Life

By the Same Author

- Secrets of Numerology
- Destiny Science and Spiritual Awakening
- Secrets of Shaktipath (Forthcoming)
- All You Wanted to Know About
  - Tantra Yoga
  - Karma Yoga
  - Jnana Yoga
  - Bhakti Yoga
  - Hatha Yoga
  - Kriya Yoga
  - Kundalini
  - Chakras and Nadis
  - Mantras
  - Dreams
  - Aura
  - Psychic Development

Academy of Kundalini Yoga and Quantum Soul

The Academy teaches the principles of Integral Path, designed by Professor Ravindra Kumar, both in theory and practice. Integral path is a scientific combination of Hatha Yoga, Karma Yoga, Jnana Yoga and Bhakti Yoga, and aims at raising the Kundalini or "dormant spiritual energy" in the practitioner in a period of about five years. With the awakening of Kundalini, a large number of dormant energy centres in the brain begin to open up and the individual acquires exceptional paranormal powers.

The Academy has a library of books from various faiths and traditions of the world. It publishes a quarterly bulletin of spiritual articles. Recently, it has started giving lessons in *Shaktipath* and prepares the students for receiving *Shaktipath Initiation* from the Guru.

SECRETS OF KUNDALINI AWAKENING
Life After Death and Quantum Soul

Ravindra Kumar, Ph. D.
Jytte Larsen, B.Com.

Academy of Kundalini Yoga and Quantum Soul

STERLING PUBLISHERS PRIVATE LIMITED

STERLING PAPERBACKS
An imprint of
Sterling Publishers (P) Ltd.
A-59, Okhla Industrial Area, Phase-II, New Delhi-110020
Tel: 26387070, 26386209 Fax: 91-11-26383788
E-mail: ghai@nde.vsnl.net.in www.sterlingpublishers.com

Secrets of Kundalini Awakening:
Life After Death and Quantum Soul

ISBN 81 207 2310 4

Published by Sterling Publishers Pvt. Ltd., New Delhi-110 020.
Lasertypeset by Vikas Compographics, New Delhi-110020.
Printed at Prolific Incorporated, New Delhi-110020.

DEDICATED TO

Inner Satguru – My High Self

Our grandmothers:
the Late Bhagwati Devi and Karen Sofie Nielsen

My Father, the Late Ganga Singh

and
Puchchi Babu – Mata

FOREWORD

In the course of my spiritual study, I have had marked episodes of activated Kundalini energy. When they first occurred, there was little in the way of literature to place these experiences into a meaningful context in my life. Even today, despite more research, this important part of our consciousness is not fully appreciated. That's why Dr. Ravindra Kumar's *Secrets of Kundalini Awakening* is such a significant work; it explains the nature of Kundalini, why it is important, and how any person can bring its benefits into his or her life. In the process of enlightening ourselves, we contribute mightily to the enlightenment of the soul of global humanity. Our ability to evolve as human beings and as souls, our ability to unite with God, our ability to leave behind forever hate, war and terrorism, will be facilitated – even determined by Kundalini.

This energy of enlightenment resides within each and every one of us, often dormant until we make the choice to seek unity with God. In our ensuing spiritual study and practice, we awaken the sleeping power within, and we are profoundly changed physically, mentally and spiritually. The hallmarks of Kundalini are phenomena such as surges of electricity in the body, detachment from the body, intense heat and fire, buzzing sounds, a feeling of being in the presence of God, and awareness of spiritual presences such as angels. More important, however, are the benefits that lie beyond the phenomena: creativity, genius, enhanced well-being, longevity, and most significant of all, enlightenment.

Experience of Kundalini have been recorded around the world since ancient times. Kundalini is the divine fire of God and the gods, the *samadhi* of adepts, the raptures of saints, the healing power that floods through the hands of healers, the inspiration of invention, the intense happiness of a peak experience. The average person may think that Kundalini belongs only to those whose spiritual practice elevates them into a rarified atmosphere of consciousness, but this is not so. Kundalini is universal, available to all. Anyone who prays or meditates reqularly is likely, at some point, to feel the power of Kundalini.

My own experiences resulted from spiritual study, meditation and intuitive/psychic development. Not knowing much about Kundalini in the beginning, I initially viewed these experiences as isolated episodes. As I learned more about Kundalini, I realised the importance of understanding its role in the development of consciousness, and of encouraging it to become more active in a gradual and productive manner.

Some years ago, I was privileged to meet Dr. Ravindra Kumar and become familiar with his work. Dr. Kumar is a man of great spiritual depth, knowledge and wisdom. Through his years of study and spiritual practise, he has to come into an understanding of Truth that he shares in the jewels of many works. This book, *Secrets of Kundalini Awakening* is a crown gem. Dr. Kumar weaves together Western and Eastern philosophy, religion, esotericism, mysticism, science and psychology, to explain from different viewpoints, the nature of the soul and the nature of reality. From his own experience, he has developed the Integral Path, a practical way for the spiritual seeker to open Kundalini and develop spiritual consciousness. Specific instructions and exercises are given throughout.

The more we know about Kundalini and how to bring in into flower within us, the more we will benefit from it, both as individuals and as part of the collective soul of humanity. Kundalini furthers our wordless understanding of the nature of creation, our part in the whole of all things, and our ultimate unity with God.

The essence of Kundalini is captured in Psalm 19, which reads in part:

> The heavens are telling the glory of God;
> and the firmament proclaims his handiwork.
> Day to day pours forth speech,
> and night-to-night declares knowledge.
> There is no speech, nor are there words;
> their voice is not heard;
> yet their voice goes through all the earth,
> and their words to the end of the world.
>
> In them he has set a tent for the sun,
> which comes forth like a bridegroom leaving his chamber,
> and like a strong man runs its course with joy.
> Its rising is from the end of the heavens,
> and its circuit to the end of them;
> and there is nothing hid from its heat.

When Kundalini is awakened through attunement to the higher planes, we are quickened in the heat of divine fire. The splendour of divine love flows through us. It is vital that we recognise the Kundalini power within, and learn how to cultivate it in the name of Truth and Love. The more we do so, the less we will descend into fear and hate. In fact, ultimately, we will not even be able to do so, for our collective soul consciousness will be firmly anchored in the light and unconditional love of the Godhead. We will truly reside in the Kingdom of God. This future will not happen, however, unless we choose it.

And in *Secrets of Kundalini Awakening*, we have an excellent guide to help us realise that choice.

Rosemary Ellen Guiley, Ph.D.
Author, *The Encyclopedia of Saints and Breakthrough Intuition*

PREFACE

There is an ocean of knowledge available in the findings of various faiths and organisations, some of which have been actively searching for "truth" for the past several millenniums and some for many centuries. I consider it a pity that the so-called modern researchers engage themselves in an independent research from scratch without looking into the knowledge that already exits elsewhere. In my opinion, the best approach would be to blend one's efforts with existing results from any source, without any prejudice and with an open mind. Each religion, each guru or each master considers its or his own path to be the only true one and talks negatively about others. If one looks carefully, one may find that the same thing may be called by a different name in another sect, and if discerned properly, it can tremendously enrich one's own findings. Furthermore, it will provide greater authenticity to one's finding, and one would be confident of one's results.

According to Hindu scriptures, *The Egyptian's Book of the Dead, The Tibetan's Book of the Dead,* The Theosophical Society, and the teachings of great souls, such as Buddha, Jesus and Mohammed, the universe has seven divisions: physical, etheric, astral, mental or psychic, spiritual, cosmic and *nirvanic*. Human consciousness is found to pass through the same seven levels, which are related to the seven *chakras* in the body, on its evolutionary journey to God. There may be some difference in arrangements according to different faiths, and certainly there are different names according to corresponding vocabularies. These levels also agree, more or less, with modern diverse authorities, such as Sri Aurobindo, Carl Jung, Osho Rajneesh and Martinus. I would further confirm their authenticity with my own experiences through meditation over the years. With the awakening of *kundalini*, one passes through these stages systematically. Witnessing the soul or *atman* as a dimensionless point of existence or awareness, experiencing God or the Absolute in one's cherished form and finally a connection with the Great Void or Nothingness – they all happen in a subjective way. There comes a "point of no return" where one has to be very careful so as not to lose one's physical existence forever.

This book is an endeavour to present all these facts, to discuss various methods of achieving cosmic consciousness and to suggest a "short path" for the awakening of *kundalini*. The journey to God has to be made alone, and the "Integral Path", which is based on the classical methods and coupled with a scientific combination, can bring results in a single lifetime. If one takes the old proverb seriously: "The man who reads is the man who leads", I can say for sure that one does not need a physical "guide", and one receives even *shaktipat* directly from God, of course, at the proper time.

If one is looking for a single factor which is responsible for an individual's genius; outstanding performances in any walk of life, such as, art, sports, drama, music, science, war, occult sciences, philosophy of life, understanding of higher laws, paranormal faculties; or being a spiritual adept of the order of a saint, then it is the "Spiritual Energy Kundalini".

Ordinarily, this power is asleep at the base of the spine, and the person is known to be an average or ordinary individual; but when this power awakens, either by accident or by sustained special efforts, then the individual is known for the "extraordinary" in him/her from that time onwards. It is the power of *kundalini* which is known to be active in most of the outstanding personalities in different fields and in different parts of the world from time immemorial.

In my first book, *Secrets of Numerology* (1992), I attempted to show that the destiny of an individual is fixed even before he/she takes birth; events simply unfolding one by one, without any control of the person on them, as if one is a puppet in the hands of some mysterious power somewhere in the universe. Great personalities, such as Abraham Lincoln, John F. Kennedy, Martin Luther King, Julius Caesar, Indira Gandhi, Mahatma Gandhi, all knew in advance intuitively about their imminent death and even the manner of dying, as stated in their own speeches; yet, they could not avoid their assassinations and the requirement of the destiny was fulfilled in each case. A method of knowing one's nature and destiny in full detail through one's name and date of birth is presented in the book.

My second book, *Destiny, Science and Spiritual Awakening* (1997) shows that the laws of science also equally apply to the human nature. Thus, Newton's second law of motion – everybody continues in a state of rest or uniform motion except in so far as it is compelled by some external force to change that state – also applies to the human destiny. The average person lives the destiny fixed in his life, unless the 'external force' of 'spiritual awakening' is applied to the course of life. A person has seven centres of energy in his body; when the *kundalini,* on awakening, crosses the third centre, the individual starts having some hold on the events of his life. As the *kundalini* crosses further centres of energy, the aspirant becomes the master of his own life and one can shape the events of his life according to his liking. In India, there is a common saying, "A yogi makes his own destiny." Spiritual awakening leads to inner peace, understanding of higher laws and finally to Self-realisation and understanding of God. The chain of death and rebirth is broken once and for all, and the person lives a liberated life on earth.

In the third book, *Journey Back to Our True Home – Through Spiritual Energy Kundalini* (1998), I have tried to show that *kundalini* is the common denominator in all religions or faiths, although the process is known by different names and the vocabulary has different terms according to different traditions and beliefs. A married person is more successful on the path of Self-realisation than a single person, since he/she has a direct encounter with the five enemies – greed, lust, anger, attachment and ego. With the passage of *kundalini* through each of the seven centres, the personality of the aspirant is gradually transformed and developed towards spiritual perfection. Powers of speech, rejuvenation and love for humanity are attained in the course. One passes through the three stages of "inner turmoil, death and resurrection". As per Lord Jesus Christ, "Only the Twice Born will enter the Kingdom of God", and this is the experience lived by a person whose *kundalini* is awakened. Regular guidance comes through dreams, according to the theory of Carl Gustav Jung. Before the awakening of the *kundalini*, the soul tries to return to earth as apparitions or as proper births through the womb of a mother because of the attraction of worldly things and relations. However, after the awakening, the soul's chain of reincarnations is broken and It proceeds to higher realms for a better life and further lessons on the path of God. A hierarchy of higher planes is also given, through which the soul gradually passes. The Integral

Path, which is a scientific combination of all systems of yoga, is presented, following which a householder can live the best possible life on earth and yet reach the Kingdom of God.

The present book, which is the fourth in the series, is an attempt to elaborate upon the knowledge of the universe and the Soul, and various methods which can be used for the awakening of *kundalini*. According to Jiddu Krishnamurti, no two persons have the same fingerprints; and as such, no two persons will have the same method for the awakening of *kundalini*. However, the adepts have laid down different procedures and it is for the individual to choose the best suited method of oneself. Guidance comes from the nature and the "Inner Satguru" from time to time – but only to that person who jumps into the path with a strong determination and with full "faith and surrender" to God Almighty.

The experiences of the soul in the universe can only be had after the death of the physical body. Nevertheless, there is a way to have these experiences before the physical death – and that is through the awakening of the *kundalini*. A person with an awakened *kundalini* sees the universe regularly as visions and out-of-body experiences. Thus, such a person experiences life after death even before dying. In fact, meditation takes an aspirant through the trio of "inner turmoil, death and resurrection", since the successful stage of meditation is an experience of death while still living in this physical body. The knowledge of beyond inspires the person to live the righteous kind of physical life on earth because then he knows that this life is not the end of everything. Grief, sorrow and torture are the results of the wrong belief that there is only one life; and because of that, the person tries to run as fast as he can to optimise the results in shortest possible time, one way or the other. Once the truth is known, the anxiety is over, peace pervades and the person lives a life which is good here and which also paves the way for a good life after death. Now he is ready to show the way to others by way of speaking, writing and providing guidance through definite steps to achieve results. Though one cannot tell the experiences, yet one can show the way about how to reach there oneself.

A description of the universe is presented in Chapter 1 which is based on the findings of various faiths, religions and organisations for several millenniums. The common finding is that there are seven divisions from the most gross physical plane on which we live to the highest realm of the Absolute: *Sat-Chit-Ananda* (Existence-Knowledge-Bliss). Knowledge in greater details has been available for the three lower planes – physical, astral and mental while the journey beyond through higher planes is more abstract. The astral and the mental planes have been elaborated upon well and these two planes are in fact the immediate concern of the people. For example, the life of a person after committing suicide, and the life of an average developed person, have specific divisions on the astral plane. The former goes to the lowest division, while the latter goes to the third division, called the "summer land". The lower division of the mental plane is the "heaven" of various religions while the upper division is the causal plane, where a causal body is formed for the first time around the soul.

In Chapter 2, an understanding of the soul or *atman* is given according to religion and also by way of science. Thoughts of two great thinkers, Sri Aurobindo and Jung, are presented on the subject, and it is shown that both of them arrived at a similar conclusion, although they differed completely in their approach. This gives strength to the definition of *atman*, which is further supported by true-life cases illustrating the power of soul. A horizontal living is necessary for existence while a vertical living is required for getting to the knowledge of the soul. Scientific evidence is compared with the otherwise known properties of the soul, and this is in accordance with the development of quantum physics. It is concluded that the evidence through quantum physics is slowly converging on the wider properties of the soul, known already through religion and personal experiences of yogis or saints.

In Chapter 3, planes of inner reality, as visualised by Sri Aurobindo and Carl Jung, are studied to come to the conclusion that the two entirely different approaches give results which are similar to the age-old findings of religions, with some variations here and there. Jung's method is that of "individuation" and Sri Aurobindo's method is that of "transformation". Their common findings are further supported by the experiences of the Danish saint Martinus. This should confirm the belief that the universe has seven clear divisions and this knowledge should help the seekers on their spiritual journey. A natural definition of *kundalini* emerges from the study.

Chapter 4 deals with various methods used in the world for opening the gateway of higher consciousness. Reasonable details of methods, beginning with the ancient Vedic approach to the modern-day techniques, are presented. In the end, it is hinted that the scientific combination of various paths in the form of "integral path" is the most useful approach and, perhaps, the shortest path to know reality. This path uses the technique of *Kundalini Yoga* which is the subject matter of the next chapter.

Chapter 5 elaborates upon the main purpose of the book, which is to present in detail the method of *Kundalini Yoga*, which, coupled with some other factors, is called the "Integral Path". The method was presented in short in my previous book *Journey Back To Our True Home*. Here, the method is elaborated in full detail, including the various yogic postures as a part of *Hatha Yoga*, chanting and prayer as a part of *Bhakti Yoga* (path of devotion), studying connected literature as a part of *Jnana Yoga* (path of knowledge) and recognising the sex-drive as a part of *Tantra Yoga*. Activities of *Karma Yoga* (path of selfless action) are automatically included. Thus, it is a balanced combination of various paths which minimises the chances of anything going wrong, and covers most of the methods of spiritual development. Various stages of transformation, through the knowledge of *nadis* and *chakras*, is presented. Various symptoms of an awakened *kundalini* are described. Different stages of the "inner journey" are discussed. Through this knowledge, an aspirant can reach the goal of Self-realisation and understand the meaning of God. A practitioner can find out the stage he is currently passing through by the recognition of the symptoms one is experiencing at present. The Integral Path is proposed to be the "shortest path" to God and the results can be achieved in a single lifetime, if everything goes well.

A bibliography for the whole book is presented at the end of the book. A glossary of words, especially the ones with a Sanskrit origin, is also presented at the end. Finally, an index is provided for ready reference.

I am grateful to my Gurus Pythagoras, Saint Asaramji, Dr. B. S. Goel and Sri Herald Klemp for the initiations and spiritual help I received from them time and again. My sincere regards are due to my mother, Mrs. Lakshmi Devi, and Mrs. Ellen Marie Andersen, for their invaluable love and blessings. Works of several worthy authors have been freely consulted by me and I wish to thank them all from the core of my heart. Useful discussions with some of my friends in the field of religion and parapsychology have helped me from time to time. Notable amongst them are Wm. Henry Belk II, Rev. Richard Luis Batzler, Dr. Claire G. Walker, Dr. John F. Miller III, Rosemary Ellen Guiley, Dr. Bonny Greenwell, Barbara Harriș Whitfield, and Dr. Rabia Lynn Clark; my thanks are due to all of them. I should record my gratitude to my brother, Jitendra Singh, my son, Atul Singh, and my daughter, Seema Singh, who have given me special love and care and who carried on the necessary work and duties whenever I was out of India.

Ravindra Kumar

CONTENTS

1

THE UNIVERSE

Introduction

Although the formal and working definition of "Kundalini" has been given earlier (Kumar 1998), we will postpone further discussions in this context, until we have acquired a reasonable knowledge of the universe and its divisions, and the properties of the Quantum Soul. Understanding the universe and its purpose will be the motivating factor to know *kundalini* and the various methods to awaken it. Thus, we now turn towards the knowledge of the universe.

The Universe

According to the Hindu philosophy (Mehta 1994, Vaze n.d.) and the knowledge gathered through the study of *The Egyptian's Book of the Dead, The Tibetan's Book of the Dead*, Theosophical Society, Eckankar, hundreds of research projects carried out in the West over a period of about 150 years, the experiences of the saints and prophets available from time to time, and a variety of near-death experience and cases of contacting the spirit of a dead friend or relative collected by J. D. Goyal (1996), the universe appears to be divided in the following "seven grand divisions".

Table 1
Seven Divisions/Planes of the Universe and Their Properties

1. Divine		*Adi*	Basic nature	Unmanifested
2. Monadic		*Anupama*	Basic nature	Manifested
3. *Atmic*		*Nirvanic*	*Sankalpa* (Will)	Spiritual
4. Intuitional		*Buddhic*	Love (Pure)	Inner-knowledge
	(*Maharlok*)	Causal-*Karana* (upper division)		
5. Mental			Thought	Analytical intellect
	(*Swarglok* or Heaven)	*Manasa*-Mental (Lower division)		
6. Astral	(*Bhuvarlok*)	*Karma* (Desire)	Sentiments	Attachment Detachment
7. Physical	(*Bhulok*)	*Sthool*	*Karma*	Sensual knowledge

Each of the seven planes is further divided into seven sub-planes; as such, we are dealing with altogether 49 sub-planes in the universe.

The earliest timeless scriptures of the Hindu philosophy – the *Vedas* and the *Upanishads* – are very well supported, verified and confirmed by the modern research of the West. The Western research is based mainly on the cases of "automatic writing", "mediums", "near-death experiences", "past-life regression" and "out-of-body experiences". Volumes of books have been written on these subjects in the last two centuries. In automatic writing, the spirit of a dead person first attracts the attention of a living person either in a dream-vision of materialised body or by throwing objects of the house here and there. And then, when the living person agrees to follow the spirit of the dead friend, relative or whatever, he takes a paper and holds a pen between the fingers and the spirit starts writing through that pen on the paper. One of the well-known books in this direction is *Raymond* written by Raymond, after he contacted his famous scientist father Sir Oliver Lodge, some time after the former passed away. Another book is *Post-mortem Journal* which was written when Lawrence of Arabia came in contact with his lady-friend and writer Jane Sherwood soon after his death. *Beyond the Horizon* was written when Mr. Gordon contacted his friend and writer, Grace Rocher, after his death. *After Death,* which has been translated in many languages and which appears in several editions, was written when W.T. Sted was in contact with his friend, Julia, after his death. *Life in the World Unseen* and *More About Life in the World Unseen* were the two books which appeared when Anthony Borgia was contacted by Monsigner Robert Hufbesnon after his death.

Several books have appeared on out-of-body experiences written authentically by their authors after a lot of research and personal experiences. Robert Monroe and Dr. Ian Stevenson are two well-known writers in this direction, in addition to several others. Monroe and Stevenson conducted hundreds of experiments on self and other subjects and described the life outside the physical body. Their findings show that the individual outside his physical body has the feelings of freedom and unconditional happiness and he does not like to return to the physical body. Furthermore, one could exist either as a male or as a female, if one wants to, while outside one's physical body, according to Monroe. A particular male always enjoyed being a female whenever outside his body. Dr. Stevenson's landmark book *20 Cases Suggestive of Reincarnation* has been followed by several others.

Hell and Heaven

There is a series of books by Stephen O'Brien (1989, 1991) of Swansea, UK, about the life in the worlds beyond.

He holds big sessions comprising several hundred people in a hall, who exchange information with their dead relatives and friends with him as the medium. O'Brien has visited the lower subdivisions of the astral plane several times and met with people who had created their own heels. With repeated efforts and great difficulty, he could pull some of them out from their self-created prisons. For example, a woman who had killed her own daughter-in-law was so self-pitied and critical of herself that she could not imagine the reality of free life. O'Brien repeatedly convinced her and brought her out of her own web and put her into a higher subdivision. This is evolution, and good souls are always eager to help those who need it. Sri Yukteshwar Giri, guru of Swami Yogananda, stated in a posthumous appearance that he (Giri) is constantly busy in helping people on the higher realm (Yogananda 1986). One is also referred to read the books on Eckankar, for example, by Paul Twitchell (1969) and Harold Klemp (1987), who have been regular visitors to different subdivisions of the astral plane and their experiences confirm the text of this paragraph. Here is a contradiction with orthodox religions which say that there are hells for sinful people to suffer after death, as for example, burning in fire, cutting of head by a saw or sinking in the pool of blood, etc. Once I visited "Tiger Garden" in Singapore which has a large section displaying varying conditions one could suffer in "hell". Perhaps, the transcendentalists tried to teach the simple-minded people in this gross way. In reality, hell is created by one's own wicked thinking. Like-minded people may group together and live in a condition of self-created hell; a finding in disagreement with orthodox religions.

In the words of Martinus (1933, 23), "This sphere is known on the physical plane as 'purgatory' and has furthermore, through superstition, been called 'hell'. There will thus be a certain unpleasant zone for all beings with imperfections to pass through after physical death. But the 'eternal fire' or 'everlasting damnation' with which the primitive imagination has quipped it certainly does not exist." According to Martinus, the individual arrives here with a mission to learn not to make mistakes, not to commit suicide or murder again, not to live unnaturally. It can be unpleasant, but it is the guide to perfect life or the direction towards God. He goes on to say that this area is only a small part of the whole spiritual zone, which otherwise constitutes an ocean of light and bliss; it is, in its most profound analysis, a divine blessing. And, there will, therefore, in reality, be no justifiable basis whatsoever for mourning the unnatural death or departure to another world of friends or relatives.

People with noble and serene thoughts are found to go to higher subdivisions, which have heaven-like conditions, though not actual heavens. Here too, like-minded people may group together and live in heaven-like conditions. Of course, there are no rivers of honey or milk, or beautiful women to be enjoyed with, as wrongly mentioned in some religions. Thus, hell and heaven have an entirely different reality than what is projected in some religions. This is also confirmed by the soul-travel experiences of several yogis, such as Yogananda (1986), Muktananda (1972), Sivananda (1991), etc.

On the Death of My Son was written by Jasper Swain of Pietermaritzburg, South Africa. Until recently, Swain was a magistrate and he had regular communications with his son who had died in an accident. In the words of Mike, the deceased son of the magistrate (Swain, 1974, 25), "As I said, thought is all-powerful here. For example, if I want to own a brand new Jaguar, all I have to do is visualise the car in my mind, and it is created right there before my eyes, out of the energy of this world." According to Mike, if two persons are far away from one another and they want to make contact, telepathy is the accepted thing there. One has to think of the fellow one wants to speak to, and bingo! He's right there. They contact each other as easily as we use the telephone, except that they do not need a telephone. If someone wants to talk to you, you first hear him in your mind. If you want to go to him, you merely exert your will and in two ticks, you're right there! As he says, it takes a bit of getting used to, but it beats TV by a mile! Everything seems to be perfect there. And again, one can travel from one end of the realm to the other as fast as lightning. There bodies never get tired. Illness and sickness do not exist there. That is a world of perfection according to Mike. The soul that inhabits our body operates like a system of electrical impulses, most people call it the 'etheric body'. The *New Testament* agrees that human personality does survive the barrier of death. Master Jesus himself revealed his etheric body to his disciples. He even showed them the nail holes in his hands. In other words, he recreated his earthly body out of etheric matter; out of the electric impulses which had activated the flesh and blood body. Being a master, he was enlightened to do so, for a master has full control of all the energy levels on the earth and can bend them all to his will. Continuing the description of the body possessed by him, Mike said, "There is quite a difference between the 'me' that lives in this world, and the 'me' that lived in your world! My body does not need food or drink to keep it going; nor does it need sleep to restore it. There are no excretory organs in our bodies. For example, when I drink a glass of water, it just diffuses itself, throughout my system, and that is what! In other words, it is converted into energy."

Mike described different levels of existence in the region. A person from the lower level finds it very difficult, if not impossible, to enter the higher level. This is because of his coarser vibrations as compared to the finer vibrations of the higher plane. Similarly, a person from the higher level can enter a lower level but he cannot stay there for long since his finer vibrations will soon start feeling uncomfortable.

C.W. Leadbeater and Madam Annie Besant had a very good knowledge of the "astral plane" gained through the "third eye" or through "astral projections". *The Other Side of Death* and *The Astral Plane* were written by Leadbeater (1933) and *Death and After* by Annie Besant (1966), which contain wonderful details of the astral plane. Several past-life therapists have also contributed towards the knowledge of the astral life. The most famous name in this context is that of Edgar Cayce. Ana Twig was a popular British medium through whom James A. Pike contacted his son Jim who had committed suicide. Pike was a well-known advocate and later he became minister of some church. He gave a scientific description of the world beyond in the book, *The Other Side*, which is quite authentic due to the unbiased view of the writer (Pike n.d.).

Leadbeater divided the universe in seven planes. In his own words, "The names usually given to these planes, taking them in order of materiality, rising from the denser to the finer, are the physical, the astral, the mental, the *buddhic* and the *nirvanic*. Higher than this are two others, but they are so far above our power of absorption that for the moment they may be left out of consideration (Leadbeater 1933, 6). The astral region, according to him, is the second of these great planes of nature – the next above (or within). Objects and inhabitant of the astral plane are real in exactly the same way as our own bodies, our furniture, our houses or monuments are real – as real as Charing Cross. And again, "In our solar system, there exist perfectly definite planes, each with its matter of different degrees of density. Some of these planes can be visited and observed by persons who have qualified themselves for the work, exactly as a foreign country might be visited and observed." (p.5) In the whole book, Leadbeater describes the life and characteristics of the astral plane which are similar but more detailed as compared to what Mike said.

Leadbeater goes on to describe the further divisions of the astral plane. According to him, an astral plane has seven subdivisions, each of which has its corresponding degree of materiality and its corresponding condition of matter. When we speak of a man rising from one plane or sub-plane to another, we do not think of him as necessarily moving in space at all, but rather as transferring his consciousness from one level to another – gradually becoming unresponsive to the vibrations of one order of matter, and beginning, instead, to answer to those of a higher and more refined order. One world with its scenery and inhabitants seems to fade slowly away from his view, while another world of a more elevated character dawns upon him in its stead. Yet, however, there is a physical dimension for each plane or a sub-plane. "Matter of all sub-planes is to be found here on the surface of the earth, but the astral plane is much larger than the physical, and extends some thousands of miles above its surface. The law of gravitation operates on astral matter, and if it were possible for it to be left entirely undisturbed, it *would* probably settle into concentric shells." (p.16)

There are a large number of "yogis" who got their *kundalini* awakened and who wrote an account of the "higher realms" based on their personal experiences over the years. Read, for example, the books by Swami Yogananda Paramahansa, Swami Muktananda, Swami Satyananda Saraswati, Dr. Ramesh Paramananda, Pandit Gopi Krishna, Dr. B. S. Goel, Swami Sivananda, Nisargadatta Maharaj, Swami Vishnu Tirtha, etc. Reference to all these books and many more, and my own experiences have been given in the second and the third books mentioned earlier (Kumar 1997 and 1998).

Reality-Beyond Seen Personally

For the last more than a decade, I have been getting first-hand knowledge of various astral sub-planes. I have always been in the lighted areas and have seen colonies, houses and living conditions similar to those on earth. The difference is that laws of physics do not apply there. People live here in their astral bodies which are similar to the physical bodies. At times, I have found myself on planes higher than astral, where you do not have any kind of body and the existence is either as a circle of light or just existence without any dimensions. There is no sun or moon there and there is no duality of any kind; for example, there is only pleasant light but no shadow of any kind at all. Such regions are called spiritual regions, which constitute three-fourths of the entire creation while one-fourth of the creation has life with some solar system like ours (Prabhupad 1987, 139). You see yourself as a dimensionless point of awareness, call it soul or *atman*. During the whole process, you see dreams too, which are in four stages as described by Jung (1964) and others. At the final stage, you see the manifestation of the Infinite in a finite form of your liking.

My father expired in September 1992 in India. In October 1995, that is, three years after his demise, I had a chance to talk to him through a medium in Charlotte, USA. A person speaking on his behalf said that he was the gatekeeper of the mansion where my father was receiving treatment, like several others over there. My father told me that he was getting a long rest after a very long time. He said that now he did not think the same way as he used to while he was on earth. He was likely to recover soon from his ailments and was likely to get a new body after some time. And then he was likely to go to a higher and more lighted area. On my asking if he had seen my grandmother, he said that he knew that she was living on a more lighted area where he cannot go but he had seen her from a distance. He wanted me to remove his belongings from the house in Delhi so that his attention was not distracted and he requested us all to release him emotionally so that he could progress well. He told me that he could meet me after 30 days in a dream if I liked, for which he had the permission. Exactly on the 30th day I found myself on some plane in my astral body, walking with and talking to my father. A few years ago, I had talked with my deceased grandmother through an Ouija board.

To read the experiences of individual souls on the astral plane, one is referred to the works of Swain (1974), O'Brien (1991), Haslop (n.d.), Borgia (n.d.), Sted (1897), Yogananda (1986), Sherwood (n.d.), Pike (n.d.), Myers (1954), Doyle (n.d.) among several innumerable others.

Near-Death Experiences

The term NDE is due to Dr. Raymond Moody who, in his book *Life After Life*, hinted on an "entity" which survives physical death. A description of life beyond given by NDEers includes "a sense of being dead, or an out-of-body experience in which they feel themselves floating above their bodies, looking down; cessation of pain and a feeling of bliss or peacefulness; travelling down a dark tunnel toward a light at the end; meeting non-physical beings who glow, many of whom are dead friends and relatives; coming in contact with a guide or Supreme Being who takes them on a life review, during which their entire life is put into perspective without rendering any negative judgements about past acts; and finally, a reluctant return to life." (Guiley 1991, 399) Barbara Harris Whitfield (1995) and Diane Globe (1993) are two writers who are personally known to me, who had similar experiences as described above, and who have given a wonderful account of life beyond after their NDEs. Other notable writers in this direction are Atwater (1988), Moody (1988), Ring (1980, 84), Ring and Rosing (1990), Grosso (1985), Sabom (1988) and Zaleski (1987).

A brief and systematic account of the life on an astral plane is attempted in the next two sections. Looking at the hierarchy of planes (Table 1) we see that the plane next to our physical plane is the "astral plane". Hence it is logical to know about the astral plane and the mode of living there so that we are on the way to understand the subtler lives above the plane of our living, which is the only plane we know at present. Although it is said that there are seven planes of existence below our physical plane where the soul passes through the stone, mineral, plant, vegetable and animal lives before graduating to the human life in this incarnation; we decide to concentrate our attention on the physical plane upwards.

Death of the Physical Body

On the physical plane, we possess a physical body and an etheric body which is similar to the physical body but it is not bound by the physical constraints. The physical body (*sthool sharira*) is made of the three densest elements of the physical world, namely, solid, liquid and gaseous. Accordingly, the body has bones, blood and gases corresponding to these three elements. The etheric body is made of four kinds of ethers (*akashic* elements) which are subtler than the three elements of the physical body. The job of the etheric double (*pranamaya kosh* or *chhaya sharira*) is to get the light-energy from the sun and pass it on to the nervous system for its nourishment. It is through this energy only that man can move the various parts of his body which are nourished and become stronger every day. At the time of death, the soul or *atman* gives up two of its bodies – physical and etheric. The etheric body cannot be seen through the physical eyes but a clairvoyant or the yogis with their divine eyes can see it. It consists of millions of pinpoints of flashing light; and the *seven centres of energy*, called *chakras*, can be seen glowing in the central line. There cannot be a greater authentic proof than the etheric body with the seven *chakras*, which we all possess, and which can be seen anytime by a clairvoyant; to show the reality of *kundalini*, which passes through these *chakras* on awakening. The etheric body is seen to hover around the place of physical body for about twelve days. This is why, perhaps, the Hindus celebrate the 12th and 17th day in a spiritual way, after the death of the person, so as to pacify this etheric body. It has been seen moving around the grave for several days. Although it does not have consciousness, yet there seems to be some kind of attraction towards the physical body.

At the onset of death, the weaker parts of the body start closing down first. And then, the life-energy which was stored by the etheric body starts moving upwards from the feet towards the head. Other parts of the body stop functioning one by one, the heart and the lungs too. Poison mixed in the blood starts showing its effect, because the life-energy which used to keep a check on it is no more. If the soul/*atman* does not want to leave the physical body due to attachment, at this stage, one suffers with pain in a strange manner. I know one of my close relatives who complained of being bitten by scorpions and snakes and he suffered with pain for almost about an hour. He said that he wanted to die but it was not happening. The death of a person at a higher age level is relatively more simple and comfortable since one is supposed to have seen the meaninglessness of life and is supposed to have conquered the five enemies (greed, lust, anger, attachment and ego) to a good extent. The yogis, who have already experienced death in meditation, leave their body so swiftly that one does not even know when it has happened. However, for an average person, the poison starts spreading slowly and a state of coma starts approaching.

In the state of coma, which is the twilight zone of semi-consciousness, the person sees his whole life like a TV serial, in which the events are shown in a retrograde manner, that is, from the present age to youth and then to childhood. It is at this stage that the soul is one's own judge for oneself. One feels happiness and bliss corresponding to the good deeds, and grief and repentance corresponding to the so-called bad deeds. One is in a state of perfect alertness, whatever one's mental condition during one's lifetime would have been, and a sort of decision is taken about the future life to be lived. Since one is in a state of pureness, a clear and unbiased decision is taken in this regard. Whatever is not necessary is dropped from the astral body, and whatever is required according to the final thoughts/sentiments, remains in the astral body; and, correspondingly, the person finds his home in the appropriate subdivision of the astral plane. Some angels or pure beings on the higher realm are also known to help the person in arriving at the choice for the next life, in accordance with the balance of *karma.* This law of nature or God is perfect and faultless. A yogi or a person with an awakened *kundalini,* perhaps, crosses this stage as a "bypass" since he has already seen his future life on one of the higher realms in the states of meditation.

After watching the film of life, the "astral body" (*sukshma sharira*) slips out of the physical body. It is said that the gateway for the detachment of the astral body is through the crown centre in the head for a person who has conquered the five enemies – greed, lust, anger, attachment and ego. For others, there my be different outlets. However, the separating astral body is linked with the physical body through a silver cord. This silver cord goes on getting thinner and thinner and is finally severed completely at the time of death. In the dream states, when the astral body is journeying into the astral planes, it is invariably linked with the physical body through this silver cord, which goes on stretching longer and longer according to the need. At the time of death, it is just severed once and for all.

The Astral Plane

At the time of the separation of the astral body, the person normally falls asleep. This sleep may extend from a few days to a few months, depending on the physical condition of the person before death. One who has been sick, sleeps longer. Dead friends and relatives of the dying person know in advance the time of death of the person and they are normally found to be around the person at the time of death. This is confirmed by the instance of my father who died in September 1992. He used to see friends of his childhood days and some relatives in their astral bodies around him during the last few days before his death. One who does not have a friend or a relative is escorted by serving volunteers from the higher realm. There are many people up there who are always eager and ready to help the departing soul.

The gross elements of desire are precipitated at this stage and the person automatically moves to that division of the astral plane (out of the seven) to which one belongs according to the sentiments. Just as there are seven divisions of the astral plane (*bhuvarlok*), from gross to subtle – downside upwards – even so the sentiments and desires of the person are separated from most gross (outside) to the most subtle (inside). The artificial control on the sentiments at the time of living is broken now and the person appears in his real form. When the sleep is broken, the person finds himself on that division of the astral plane which vibrates with the same frequency as his precipitated sentiments/desires. Thus, a social worker or a politician who was outwardly serving others but inwardly living a selfish life with a narrow mind, will find himself on the second plane from the bottom. One's selfishness and narrow-mindedness is grosser than the subtle sentiments of helping others, and consequently, one finds oneself on the second plane. There one lives till one finds freedom from the selfish and narrow views and then moves automatically to the third or fourth sub-plane. In the physical life, such a person may be living in a very big and comfortable house, but his narrow views bring him to the lower plane of narrowness. Comparatively, a person who was living in an ordinary house in the physical world but was unselfish and a server of humanity will find him directly on the third subdivision.

The lowest or the first subdivision, thus, may be corresponding to the most selfish and brutal people who might have committed heinous crimes and who are full of animalistic desires. Since like attracts like, this plane is full of such people only, who live with their narrow and selfish mentality and are never happy. So a morose atmosphere prevails there and may be called the nearest approximation to hell. A hell which is pictured in various religions, where people are tortured in various ways, is only a manufacture of the pundits of various religions and far from reality, as mentioned earlier. Perhaps the early saints wanted to give a physical shape to the lowest subdivision for the understanding of common people who cannot have abstract imaginations. It is well that one understand the reality now.

Unselfish people, artists, writers, poets, scientists, doctors, musicians, social reformers, religious people, metaphysicians, etc., who are engaged in the service of the humanity in one way or another, would normally find themselves on one of the higher subdivisions, say from the third to the seventh, depending on their level of consciousness, after their death. The finer the thoughts, the higher the subdivision. People from the lower subdivisions gradually move to the higher subdivisions after graduating themselves from their narrow and self-confining views. A person from the lower subdivision cannot see properly the form of a person on the higher subdivision, since his gross senses cannot comprehend the subtler and finer forms of the person on the higher subdivision. On the other hand, a person from the higher subdivision can very well see and even visit a person at the lower subdivision, although he may not like to stay there for long. This is because his vibrations do not feel comfortable on the lower plane which has coarser vibrations. A person form the lower plane may go to the higher plane for a short while, but he cannot stay there for long because his vibrations cannot find a comfortable adjustment there. A person from the higher plane may not be so unhappy at the lower plane as a person of the lower plane itself, who is suffering from the coarse and faulty atmosphere there.

For some initial period, the people on the astral plane may not believe that they are dead. Or, they may like to visit their friends and relatives on the earth due to attachment. For either reason, they may come to the earth in their astral bodies and try to live the physical life and may try to talk to their loved ones. They call the person by his name but there is no response. Sometimes when this happens, you get a faint feeling that someone is calling you although you do not see the person. After repeated failures in getting the response from the living person, the astral inhabitant gets convinced that he is dead and returns to the astral plane. Normally, one is accompanied by a guide from the astral plane. A large number of cases of this kind have been described in detail by Martin and Romanowski (1991) in *We are Not Forgotten.*

People make houses and colonies on the astral plane similar to those on the physical plane. And this happens just through the power of thought. You imagine a house in all its details, concentrate on it for a while and the house is there in front of you. You imagine a car, concentrate on it and its there. You decorate the house with curtains, furniture, carpets, cutlery, etc. of your choice just by the power of thoughts. You imagine a dress of your choice, and it is there on your body. When you like to drink tea, imagine a tea-set, the tea of your liking, the table and chairs and they are all there. It is after some time that you realise the futility of all these things. You do not really need a house to live, a car to move and so on. You think of a person anywhere on the plane and you are just there with him or her. This you may call to be the conditions of the heaven since everything appears approachable. Yet there is no heaven as described by various religions. Heavens of scriptures are again the fantasies of the religious pundits. However, you still have the constraints of the astral body which suffers with the good and bad effects of desires. It is the next higher plane above the astral plane where you cease to have the astral body and then there is no cause for suffering anymore. This happens after the second death, which we are going to discuss a little later.

A person, with an awakened *kundalini* and living in the earthly world, has regular visits to various subdivisions of the astral plane. It is the fore-knowledge of the higher realms which an aspirant gets as a part of his learning, from nature or God. See, for example, the books by Yogananda (1986), Muktananda (1972), Aurobindo (1989), Gopi Krishna (1975) and several others mentioned in Kumar (1998).

Telepathy, telekinesis, levitation, precognition, clairvoyance and other ESP (extra sensory perception) powers are natural tools of life on the astral plane. Sometimes they infiltrate on the physical plane and are exhibited through certain persons. Duke University in North Carolina has been conducting research on these subjects since 1920 under the direction of Professor J.B. Rhine who expired a few years ago. Although these phenomena are reproduced in the laboratory, it has not been possible to fit any physical or mathematical model to any one of them. It can never be possible since you cannot contain the "infinite" in a "finite" frame. However, they give you a glimpse or taste of the astral plane while you are still on the physical plane. And, of course, they motivate you to live the life of a yogi so that you can say goodbye to this physical plane forever and become the inhabitant of the astral plane or even a higher plane of the spiritual nature.

A good example of the powers of astral plane being used on the physical plane is the creation of thought forms. Alexandra David Neel (1931) lived in India and Tibet for about twenty years and she participated fully in the *tantric* rituals along with a regular practice of yoga and meditation. Through the power of thoughts, she created a monkey (*tulpa*) who could be her companion and helper. For some years, it really provided her with the help and company. However, after some time it developed its own individuality and refused to obey her totally. Slowly, he became a headache for her and with great difficulty she was able to dislodge him. One can now imagine the creation of goddess Durga by gods through the collective power of thoughts, who could fight the demons and save the good gods. And again, the Psychic Being (Aurobindo 1989) or the High Self (Jung 1964) created by the soul over a series of earthly incarnations can now be understood. This Psychic Being has an individuality of its own and is the most benevolent factor bridging the gap between the soul and God.

In old age, the organs of a person become weak, and he does not have the youthful physical form, and his senses also weaken. However, on arrival at the astral plane all these defects are removed. The person lives in his youthful body, he never feels tired, hungry or thirsty. Sometimes, a defective part in his body lingers on in his memory. Such a person is placed in a mansion, which may be called a hospital, somewhere on the fifth division of the astral plane, where he is given rest and the defective part is cured gradually. It is purgatory, a station on the way. A person's way of thinking, sentiments and knowledge, attained in the physical world, remain exactly the same.

Power, position, money and honour – they all come to an end on the astral plane. Only the purity of heart, love and goodwill matter there and on the basis of these things alone one is respected. Simple and neglected people on earth, who were in fact pure and spiritual, get higher subdivisions on the astral plane and are highly respected. A person who leads the life of purity and spirituality has his soul body (causal body) looking very beautiful and lustrous. Such a person normally goes to the third subdivision after death, the place often called the "summer land." (Haslop n.d., Ivor James 1996) This place is studded with mountains, attractive gardens, river and lakes. Houses are surrounded with beautiful flowers of unearthly colours and these flowers never lose their attractiveness. There are no rains, thunderstorms or such things which might mar the atmosphere. Someone called it earth without all its negative attributes, such as, fear, jealousy, competition, selfishness, etc. According to Ivor James (1996), it cannot be a replica of earth, which is degenerate. Poets and writers on earth have been getting a glimpse of such places in their trance before writing as can be seen in the works of famous people. "Who says we are dead? It is the worldly people who are in fact dead (or asleep), because all of them live in a state of strange confusion which is very far from reality. ...A person who has no desires on the astral plane, gets everything over there. This is a paradox." (Pike n.d.)

After coming in contact with saint of "Higher Souls" and further evolution, the inhabitants of the "summer land" begin to have feelings from the realm of spiritual mind, and a feeling of restlessness to enter new experiences creeps into their consciousness. After going through a condition of temporary coma, the person awakens in the fourth or fifth subdivision or still a higher one, according to the degree of perfection. Nature is more beautiful in these higher divisions and the vibrations are more refined and subtle. Learned people, artists, poets, scientists and others of this kind make their homes here.

New senses of feeling and experiencing begin to develop on the astral plane, according to the virtues in the person. One can see and feel according to one's development. Feelings of the heart cannot be hidden from others, because they immediately convert into colours around the astral body. Thus, one naturally lives a pure and non-schizophrenic life; all dealings are straightforward, unlike those on the earth. Those who think only about themselves (on earth plane) can never be happy here (on astral plane). Such people are found to be poorest in the astral world. On the other hand, large-hearted and compassionate people live the best life here. On lower subdivisions, people continue with the worldly habits, such as, eating, drinking, etc., for quite some time, until they understand the futility of it. On higher subdivisions, people are free from such habits and they live more worthwhile life, leading towards spiritual perfection. You dress the way you like, just through the power of thoughts – you think and imagine, and you are dressed. If you wish to meet someone, just like that or for some help, the other person knows telepathically about it immediately, and you see him approaching you. Good souls can easily move from one place to another, while the lower ones remain confined to their own areas. Except for the two lower subdivisions, all other subdivisions are beautiful and fully lighted. Solid, liquid and gaseous elements can be converted into each other just by thinking. One can change one's face or shape according to one's will. However, one can recognise the other by external make-up or movements through intuition.

The physical plane has three dimensions – length, breadth and depth. The astral plane has four dimensions; the fourth dimension is said to be time, according to some scientists. Distance and time have no limitations on the astral plane. Time, having no limitations, means that a certain thing which was, which is and which will be, can all be seen at the same time. In other words, things of the astral plane have a permanent value, they have no duality or changeability. Events to happen cast their shadows in advance. That is why the friends and relatives of a dying person know in advance the time of death of the person and that is why you find them always around the dying person, a few days before he dies. The fourth dimension also implies that you can see outside as well as inside a box. You can read a book placed in the almirah without taking it out.

The situation, in the above paragraph, can be understood as follows. A person standing on top of a 50-storeyed building can easily see a procession which is going to pass through the base of the building after half an hour, while a person standing on the ground floor can neither see it nor know about it. This is an analogical understanding of the fore-knowledge of events. To understand the other situation, imagine a person who lives in and knows only two dimensions. He does not have the concept of height or depth. Suddenly if he is placed in a situation with three dimensions, he will just be baffled, he would not know what is happening. The same is the situation when a person with life in three dimensions only, happens to be in the four-dimensional space. The five senses of a man in the physical world have their limitations, they are not adequate enough to understand the reality of the astral plane. Increasing this analogy to 10, 20 or 100 dimensions, where God is, you can understand how difficult it is to understand Him through the limitation of just five senses. You need yoga and meditation which can develop extra senses necessary for the understanding of the secrets of the universe.

The astral plane has vast libraries, innumerable books on all possible subjects and unbelievable research facilities. Researchers can continue their work either on earthly or astral matters, with great satisfaction.

The usual concept of time having gone, time is now measured in the form of experiences only. The period one spends on the astral plane may vary from five years to five hundred years to five thousand years, depending on the experiences of the person, which are necessary either for the next worldly incarnation or for moving upwards to the "mental plane".

A word about the "grey world", a state suspended between the physical and astral planes. Life here can be very troublesome and indefinite since the person belongs nowhere. People who have a narrow view, who have lived a selfish and dry life, which has been full of criminal and heinous acts on earth, are surrounded by a tense and saddened atmosphere, together with innumerable people of the same kind. Even at this stage, if they do not repent for their low deeds, they slip into this "grey world". The atmosphere here is dimmer and darker. However, one is not condemned here forever. As soon as the awakening strikes, there is always a good soul to help and the person is uplifted to a higher subdivision. A sincere call never goes unheard here.

Accidental Death and Suicide

This is the subject which needs special attention because of the increasing number of cases in the world. A case of sudden death is much different from that of natural death due to either old age or long illness, in which case the desires of a person become naturally weak, and attachment with the world gets reduced considerably, which takes him to a good subdivision on the astral plane. In case of sudden death, the person is not prepared at all and worldly desires of the basic nature remain clinging to him as a natural consequence. This leads him to the lowest division of the astral plane.

There are two kinds of people in this category – those who have been living a pure and generous life; and those who have been living a life full of selfishness, anger, terror and animalism for self-satisfaction. Persons of the first category remain forgetfully and peacefully asleep, and some day when they are awakened by some good soul, they move upwards. Persons of the second category remain fully alert in this dark and dense subdivision and they become a source of trouble for everyone. For the satisfaction of their animal and unsatisfied desires, they enter the body of an angry person, intoxicated with mercilessness, or a person who is ready to do anything for the satisfaction of his low bodily desires. They try to fuel the sentiments of that person and encourage him to do the worst possible things to others. They assume a very ghastly form. Such people easily lure simple persons to do bad things. However, they are ineffective on persons of good ethics and character, and only when someone is driven towards doing a lowly act, he proves harmful. Such people can be clairvoyantly seen around the prostitution areas, butchery shops and bars or pubs.

Those who commit suicide, have planned it for some time and the scheme gets well set in their memory. Then they repeat this drama again and again for several years. A girl who committed suicide by jumping into the Thames river was found to repeat the whole show for about 20 years. According to A.P. Senate, the time and equipment were the same as those at the time of the actual suicide.

Suicide is one act which has been almost unanimously condemned by everyone. According to Eckankar, "It's my understanding that if you commit suicide, it will haunt you in your next life. You will have more misery than ever." (Klemp 1992, 46) Shri Shirdi Sai Baba said, "You must enjoy the fruit, good or bad, of your past actions; if the enjoyment be incomplete, suicide will not help you. You have to take another birth and suffer again. So instead of killing yourself, why not suffer for some time and finish up your store of the fruit of past deeds and be (done) with it once and for all?" (Rao n.d., 24) In the words of Leadbeater (1933, 77), "The position of the suicide is further complicated by the fact that this rash act has diminished the power of the ego to withdraw its lower portion into itself, and therefore has exposed him to various additional dangers; but it must be remembered that the guilt of suicide differs considerably according to its circumstances, from the morally blameless act of Seneca and Socrates through all degrees down to the heinous crime of the wretch who takes his own life in order to escape from the entanglements into which his villainy has brought him; and the position after death varies accordingly." The opinion of Martinus (1933, 22-23) is, "For the individual who commits suicide, the unpleasantness is further increased by the dreadful disappointment that death is not, as he had believed, a deliverance from his difficulties, but that he, on the contrary, in addition to being still fully conscious of them has now also inflicted upon himself the suffering that he will, to a certain extent, have to endure, and an abnormal spiritual existence with the prospect of a repetition of these difficulties in his next physical life on earth. He thus witnesses the fact that he cannot run away from his fate. Had he put up with those difficulties until death had occurred of its own accord, his spiritual existence would at least have been more normal, and strengthening for his next terrestrial life." Condemnation of suicide agrees with the teachings of almost all religions.

Although a definite layout of the subdivisions of the astral plane can never be made, yet an approximate situation can be described as follows:

Table 2
Layout of the Subdivisions of the Astral Plane in the Order of Increasing Consciousness, from below upwards

No. of Sub-division		Certain salient features
7th sub-plane	:	Heavenly worlds, yet only astral, much balanced karma, real heaven on next plane
6th sub-plane	:	More refined/advanced, fantastic landscapes, artistically/philosophically developed
5th sub-plane	:	Brighter, healing and spiritual development, churches, schools and libraries
4th sub-plane	:	Fully lighted area, grander physical surrounding, celestial beauty, nice for children
3rd sub-plane	:	First lighted area "summer land", benevolent people and good living conditions
2nd sub-plane	:	Less dark, less dense, highly materialistic people, not believing being dead
1st sub-plane	:	Dark, dense and difficult for living, bad souls looking for satisfaction through others
Grey World	:	State suspended between astral and physical planes, unrepentant hardened criminals
Physical Plane	:	Living with senses, creation and dissolution of karma, real opportunity for evolution

Grey World: A state suspended between the physical and astral plane, abode of the criminals and doers of heinous acts who are not ready to repent for their lowliest activities.

First/Lowest Sub-Plane: Dark, dense, difficult for living, comparable to the condition of a man required to live in the centre of the mountain. Abode of hardened criminals with heinous acts, dreadful creatures, cruelty, animal-man, depravity. Conditions described by all religions as orthodox hell (with the difference that it is created by the person himself by his own mentality). *Pretlok* of Hindus, where the "bad souls" are looking to enter the bodies of others for their satisfaction of base desires. Realm of astral world where animal consciousness works. Thought-forms of hundreds of millions of people charged with *prana* (life energy), created by subhuman minds due to anger, hatred, depression, etc. These thought-forms are like clouds which do affect people with similar thinking on earth adversely by providing stimulation to them. The clouds disintegrate after a while.

Second Sub-Plane: Less darker, less denser. More refined than the first. Abode of highly materialistic people. Souls who awaken here after sudden death do not have an idea that they are dead. Persons caught in in-between states. Victims of the 1914-18 war still looking for someone to kill. Great wands of loving souls to help poor creatures come out of the psychic shock and created conditions. People are taken from here to the "nursing homes" situated on the fifth sub-plane.

One should remember that each sub-plane has further seven subdivisions each or even more than that. Each of the first and the second sub-planes may thus be having innumerable souls on different subdivisions according to their states of consciousness and variations. Accordingly, the highest subdivision of the second sub-plane may be having people who are much refined and ready to move to the next sub-plane which is the first lighted area from below.

Third Sub-Plane: First "lighted area" of the astral plane, called the "summer land" by many writers. Those who have lived a good life, not necessarily religious but benevolent, not causing harm to anyone; they awaken here and they may think that they have come to paradise. It may appear to be a copy of the earth without its negative attributes. It has mountains, lands, rivers, lakes, houses, streets and gardens similar to earth, giving a feeling of familiarity. Artistic, realisation of the dreams of perfection, buildings glowing and even minerals having a participation in life. Some say that flowers also assume a human form at times here. However, according to Ivor James (1996), it cannot be the replica of earth since earth is degenerate. People live in a similar atmosphere as on earth and with the same habits of eating, drinking, dressing, travelling, meeting friends and relatives etc., everything materialising through the power of thoughts immediately. As the soul grows further and finds interaction with high souls and saints, it passes through a sudden coma before finding it awake in the fourth or the fifth sub-plane, or even a higher one, according to its consciousness.

Fourth Sub-Plane: Fully lighted area with finer vibrations than the third plane, better physical surroundings and more beautiful things. This division has a special place for children and they are looked after properly here. (Haslop n.d.)

Fifth Sub-Plane: Nicely lighted, higher vibrations, perhaps the most important division from the activity point of view. Far more beautiful, luminous, all heavens created by the minds of all religions, streets of Jerusalem, hunting grounds of Red Indians, etc., churches, schools, religious and philosophical bodies. Religious bodies congregate; they believe they are the only ones saved, happy and rewarded. Many spiritual guides of people on earth have their homes here. However, the teachers are not really great and there is a language barrier – communication is through the medium. People appear in the prime of their life here, bodies becoming younger and perfect. Books, libraries, centres of research – thousands of souls engaged in research on either astral or earthly subjects. For any particular study, the facilities available are unbelievable. People are unaware of the passing of the time. They think there is nothing better than what they have here, it is the end of everything. Learned people, artists, scientists, great persons, saints – they all belong to this region. Hospitals for reviving souls and providing them with new bodies are all here.

However, higher conditions still appeal to the intellectuals and they realise that this is only a station. From the realm of spiritual mind, they get ideas, and after a temporary coma, they may move to the sixth or seventh division.

Sixth Sub-Plane: Very well-lighted, similar to the fifth plane, still higher vibrations, much more refined, more advanced, highly developed artistically or philosophically, fantastic landscapes and so on.

Seventh Sub-Plane: Heavenly worlds, yet only astral, since the real heaven lies on the next plane – the mental plane, called *devachan* in Sanskrit.

One may live for thousands of years on the higher subdivisions since the conditions are perfect and there is no counting of time. The astral world does not have physical dimensions and it does not revolve around any physical sun like the earth does. Hence, one has to learn only through spiritual advancement that this is not the real heaven. The "second death" takes place and the astral body dies. One awakens on the lower mental plane, called the heaven or *swarglok*.

The Mental Plane

For the inhabitants of the astral plane, there is a time, when, from the realm of the spiritual mind, comes a feeling of restlessness to enter new experiences. The astral body begins to die and the person awakens in his spiritual body in the spiritual world called *devachan*. This is the "second death" the person undergoes and it is the transition from the "astral plane" to the "mental plane". While on earth, the soul lives in a "physical body" made of physical elements (earth, water, fire, air and ether), while on the astral plane, it lives in the "astral body" made of astral atoms having finer vibrations compared to earth, and while on the mental plane, it has the "mental body" made of atoms having still finer vibrations. One can see and feel better, and one feels like a butterfly which is beautiful and light.

The mental plane has two divisions, the lower division is the "heaven" (*swarglok*) while the upper division is the "causal plane" (*maharlok*). This is the actual heaven described by all religions where the person reaps the harvest of his good *karma*. It is the astral body which responds to the desire (*kama*) resulting in attachment/detachment or the good/bad. Since this body has already been shed, one is out of all dualities and the person lives in complete happiness and bliss. No words can describe the feelings there. However, there are no rivers of milk or honey flowing here, and no beautiful fairies to give you physical pleasures. It was only an imagination or concoction of the priests of various religions. On lower division or heaven, the soul has a "mental body", while on upper division or *maharlok*, the soul has a "causal body". The causal body is the *first manifested form around the soul*, that is, the beginning of a body with form for all time to come, as long as the soul lives in the lower worlds below the causal plane. Above the causal plane, the soul journeys by itself, without any form or body around it.

In the words of Sri Yukteshwar Giri (Yogananda 1986), "I live in that part of the astral plane which is known as *Hiranyalok*. I help many developed soul coming from earth, in getting freedom. People here are free from the problems of eating, drinking, etc. One can meet here with one's mother, father, son, daughter, wife or husband, etc. not only from the previous life, but from several lives before the previous one. One is free from untimely death, disease and old age. It is the only institution which works out everything here. One only needs the will here to accomplish anything or everything." Sri Yukteshwar said the above words through his "materialised temporary body" some time after his physical death, using his yogic power. The *Hiranyalok* talked about by Sri Yukteshwar is perhaps the *swarglok* (heaven), since he said about moving to the "causal plane" from there. He also said about staying in the *Hiranyalok* for a long time, which is possible in *swarglok* (heaven) only. And again, according to many others too, one can meet with relatives of the previous life on the astral plane, but the relatives from several other lives can be met with only in the *swarglok* (heaven)." (Goyal 1996)

I had a chance to talk to Guru Kirpal, through a medium in North Carolina, for about an hour. He told me that he was living on the "mental plane" and there were many saints and highly evolved souls who were living on that plane. Sri Yukteshwar Giri was also living on the mental plane. It suggests that most of the Self-realised souls live on the mental plane and help people on the lower planes in the process of their evolution. These high souls can talk to other souls and even travel to lower planes for interactions.

To understand the interpenetration of the various planes into each other, let us look at the following example: Take a bottle and fill it up with water, sand, ash and some pieces of stone. Shake it and then put it on the table. After a while you will see that the heaviest pieces of stone have settled down near the bottom and the lighter ones are on top of them, according to the order of their weight. Above the stones you will see the particles of sand and then the ash and on top of everything you will find water. Water being the lightest of all, it is at the highest region where no other matter can remain; and at the same time water is found in every division of the bottle. Similarly, ash is the next element, and in that region, sand and stones are not found; but at the same time ash is also seen in every lower division of the bottle. So the second division has two elements – water and ash. Next, you will find sand, ash and water, but no stones, in the third division. And in the fourth division, you will see all the four elements – water, ash, sand and stones. Even so, the highest and first "divine plane" has only divine elements in it. The second "monadic plane" has divine and monadic elements in it. The third "*atmic* plane" has divine, monadic and *atmic* elements in it. The fourth "intuitional plane" has divine, monadic, *atmic* and intuitional elements in it. The fifth "mental plane" has divine, monadic, *atmic,* intuitional and mental elements in it. The sixth "astral plane" has divine, monadic, *atmic,* intuitional, mental and astral elements in it. And the seventh and the last "physical plane" has all the seven elements in it – divine, monadic, *atmic*, intuitional, mental, astral and physical.

As a person evolves from the physical to the astral plane, he leaves the physical elements behind and is now made of the upper six elements only. When he further evolves from the astral to the mental plane, astral elements are also given up forever, and the person possesses only mental, intuitional, *atmic*, monadic and divine elements. On further evolution, he says goodbye to the mental elements too, and the constitution is now made up of intuitional, *atmic*, monadic and divine elements. On further evolution, he says goodbye to the mental elements too, and the constitution is now made up of intuitional, *atmic*, monadic and divine elements only. On reaching the atmic plane, he is made of *atmic*, monadic and divine elements only. On the monadic plane, he possesses only the monadic and divine elements. And finally, when the highest order saint merges into the divine and becomes one with Him, he does not have even the monadic elements and is made purely of the divine elements, truly in the image of God Himself. Monad being the first manifestation from the divine source, its extinction means the unmanifested Self in the divine realm of God. However, just as water has an approach to all the lower divisions of the bottle, even so, the divine person has an approach to all the lower planes.

One can visualise all the seven planes in a circular form round the physical plane, just like the peels of an onion in circular layers, one above the other, each plane penetrating its elements in all the lower ones.

Seven planes are divided into seven subdivisions each, making 49 subdivisions altogether. Out of these 49, the last two, 49th-solid and 48th-liquid, constitute the visible world, which can be seen through the physical eyes; the rest of the 47 elements constitute the invisible world, which can be seen through clairvoyant eyes only. The 49th plane has all the 49 elements in it, from solid to the divine. The 48th plane does not have the solid element in it but it has all the other 48 elements in it, from liquid to the divine. The 47th plane does not have the last two elements – solid and liquid – in it, but it has all the remaining 47 elements in it, from air to the divine. And so on and so forth.

Spirit individualised becomes a soul. Its beginning is the original and biggest secret of all times. Thus, the soul or *atman* is an element of God and this element, in its original form, remains established and present on the "monadic plane". In its original form, it is pure and uninvolved. When the ray of this element descends into the lower plane, the attributes of that plane gather around it. When it descends to the next lower plane, attributes of the second lower plane make the second cover (of its attributes) around the soul. Descending on the third plane, the third cover of attributes envelopes the soul. Proceeding in this manner, when the soul reaches the lowest or seventh "physical plane", it has in it the attributes of all the seven planes as various layers or covers around itself. On the "journey back home", these layers or covers are removed one by one and the soul shines again in its original form. How to achieve this is the subject matter of the later part of this book.

The "personality" of an individual is the group of four lower bodies – mental, astral, etheric and physical. Etheric body surrounds the physical body as an aura that can be seen by a clairvoyant. Many times the etheric double, which is a replica of the physical body, is seen hovering surround the cemeteries for a few days after physical death. This group is a perishable one, and it is formed around the basic body, called the "causal body", which is made through the elements of the upper division of the mental plane, called the "causal plane" or *maharlok*. The causal body is the personal carrier of the soul and it is imperishable. It is the centre of creation and a storehouse of unmanifested and abstract thoughts. Experiences of the individual from the previous lifetimes remain stored in the causal body in "seed form"; and every time the person reincarnates, these seeds of experiences gathered so far blossom like flowers. Since the causal body is made of pure *atmic* elements, it stores only the virtues collected so far, such as, tolerance, forgiveness, compassion, humility, devotion, courage, capacity of and perfection in work, wisdom, intuitive knowledge, etc. In each successive reincarnation, these virtues get compounded and in a particular incarnation they appear as an "integral part of the nature" of the person. Negative attributes, such as weaknesses, vice, corruption, selfishness, exploitation, covetousness, self-gratification, etc., do not find a place in the causal body because of the purity of its elements. However, the personality which is made of mental, astral, etheric and physical bodies stores the weaknesses and shortcomings of the person which do manifest in successive incarnations, in some form or another. For example, a person who might have broken one of his legs in the previous life, is found to have insufficient strength in that particular leg in the present incarnation. The astral body, which is a produce of the *kamalok* (plane of desires), stores in itself the weaknesses of the person, which are added to the causal body. But they fade away with the death of the personality and the causal body, while the virtues remain till the end.

There are two kinds of thoughts – manifested and abstract. An average person, who constitutes the majority of humanity, can contemplate on thoughts with forms only, abstract thinking is not his arena. This means that an average person does not contemplate on ideal thoughts like tolerance, forgiveness, compassion, humility, devotion and the like. Accordingly, an average person has his reach only up to the lower division of the mental plane, called heaven or *swarglok*, which is the arena of manifested forms. The highest amongst such people are perhaps the followers of the so-called religions and different faiths, social reformers, etc. They believe God to have a human form and living in heaven. Their final reach and ultimate ambition is to reach heaven and to enjoy the good life there. The religion tells them that they will be the playmates of God and that they will have all kinds of pleasures, which have their limitations on earth. They believe that all limitations will be removed in heaven and they will enjoy new things every day on a permanent basis. This is the climax of thoughts in the manifested form – there is nothing beyond it, as they believe, and they actually stop there. It is said that exhaustion of good *karmas* brings them back to the lower worlds in new incarnations. And this cycle keeps repeating endlessly. Even if the cycle is not repeated, they may live forever in the heaven (lower mental plane) – and that is the end of everything.

The second category; which is a very small part of the humanity, say, ten per cent at its best, is that of the abstract thinkers, such as artists, psychologists, doctors, professors and researchers in various fields of study. Such people can have an experience of the next higher division of the mental plane, called the causal plane or *maharlok*. They have their reach to this world of abstract thoughts.

Beyond the mental plane is the reach of those persons who can be called "really religious", who contemplate on "God without attributes", that is, *Nirguna Brahman*, or those who are abstract thinkers of the level on which they begin to get "intuitive wisdom" from beyond. They belong to the "intuitional or *buddhic* plane". And above the intuitional plane is the approach of the persons who have either contemplated on the *atman* or the *soul*; or who through their regular metaphysical or yogic/meditational practices have realised the High Self (of Jung) or the *Atman* (of Hindus) or *Ruha* (of Sufis) or the Light of the Void (of Buddha) or the Father (of Jesus Christ). They belong to the "*atmic* plane", the plane of *nirvana* or liberation, which provides the freedom from the false and which breaks the bonds of "reincarnations" or the "cycle of death and rebirth" forever. Selective people from all religions have reached this stage. [See, for example, my book *Journey Back To Our True Home* (Kumar 1997)] This region is composed of exceptionally beautiful mountains, landscapes, rivers, trees, fruits, flowers, and is lighted equally everywhere without an obvious source.

You see yourself as a *dimensionless point of awareness,* moving freely with the speed of thoughts, if and when you want; having no hunger, thirst, or desire for sex, etc., in a state of perpetual bliss, incomparable to any kind of pleasure on earth, having an ability to see in all directions, and having such an intuitive knowledge of everything that you do not want to know anything at all. You have an intutitive belief that you always existed and you will always exist. This is the state of *Sat-Chit-Ananda,* that is, *Existence-Knowledge-Bliss,* which are the attributes of Brahman or God Absolute. Since the soul (*atman*) is akin to God (*Paramatma*), you get the intuitive understanding of God. Thus Self-realisation leads to God-realisation intuitively. Such a person does not have any requirement on earth; one is not interested to know the past, nor is interested in speculating about the future, and, of course, is unconcerned about the present. One moves as a self-contented and liberated person around the globe, always happy and cheerful.

Experiencing a higher plane sitting on a lower plane does not mean that you travel bodily to that plane. In fact, the higher plane is experienced right there where you are sitting. It is the consciousness that transforms from the lower to the higher level. Consider, for example, the experiment with the bottle having water, ash, sand, and stones. Sitting at the bottom of the bottle you will see only the stone or sand if your consciousness is vibrating with thoughts of a solid, and you will see only the water if your consciousness is vibrating with thoughts of a liquid, although both stone and water are present at the same place. Similarly, the physical plane has elements from all the planes, but you will live the reality of only that plane corresponding to which your consciousness is vibrating. Thus, a clairvoyant is living the reality of the astral plane although he is sitting on the physical plane. A saint is living the reality of the mental plane or the *atmic* plane, according to the development of his consciousness, although he is sitting only on the physical plane. However, after the death of the physical body, one may be transferred bodily to the region of the astral plane; or to the mental plane directly, if one's physical and astral bodies have died simultaneously. One finds a permanent abode on that plane after death for which one has qualified oneself by raising one's consciousness. After all, the vast universe has different layers with varying densities, representing various planes, and the Creator would like all of them to be inhabited by proper beings. And this is what happens.

The following table gives the distribution according to the Hindu philosophy:

Table 3

S. No.	Plane (Lok) (According to Hindu Scriptures)	Plane (Lok) (According to Knowledge of Brahman)	Attributes of the Plane	Body According to the Plane
1.	*Golok*	*Adi lok*	Attributeless God *Nirguna Brahman* (unmanifested)	
2.	*Vaikunth lok*	Monadic *lok*	Basic nature (manifested)	Monad (Spark of God)
3.	*Satya lok* (Plane of truth)	*Atmic lok*	*Atmic* elements	*Atman* (Will, action, intellect)
	Tap lok (Plane of austerities)			
4.	-------- *Jnana lok* (Plane of wisdom)	*Buddhic lok*	Para/Inner wisdom	*Anandamaya kosh* (Plane of intuition)
	Maharlok (Causal plane)		Abstract Thoughts	*Vigyanamaya kosh* *Karana sharira* (Causal body)
5.	------- *Swarglok* (Heaven)	*Manasik lok*	--------------	*Manasik sharira* (Mental body)

6. *Bhuvarlok* (Astral plane)	Astral *lok* (Mental plane)	Thoughts with forms Artistic, compassionate, benevolent, Properties of: Purity, activity and rigidity (*satogun, rajogun* and *tamogun*)	*Sukshma sharira* or *Vasana sharira* (Astral body)
7. *Bhulok* (Physical plane)	*Sthool lok*	Memory, light, life, activity, gaseous, liquid, solid,	*Pranamaya kosh* (etheric double) --------- *Annamaya kosh* (Physical body)

A natural question to ask, at this juncture, would be: what is the duration of stay of a person on the astral plane? Well, it is a difficult question to answer, nevertheless, there is some information available, which is based on research. The length of stay on a plane depends on the stage of evolution one has reached and one's state of mind. Artists, scientists, philosophers, poets and writers, and the followers of spiritual path spend the least time on the astral plane (less than ten years) and maximum time in the heaven (several hundred years). Honest, ideal thinkers of justice, mental workers, social reformers, humanitarians, philanthropic and religious persons may spend a few tens of years on the astral plane and a few hundreds of years (around five hundred) on the lower mental plane. Those who do not think ill of others, average citizens and believers in religion may live for fifty to sixty years on the astral plane and two to three hundred years on the *swarglok*. Medium workers and businessmen, narrow-minded and selfish people may live for less than hundred years on the astral and up to around two hundred years or so on the lower mental plane. Superstitious and physical labourers may spend up to around a hundred years on the sixth plane (astral) and they might visit the fifth plane (mental) for a short period in a subconscious state of mind. Barbarians, lazy and uneducated people are normally expected to spend around a hundred years or so on the sixth plane (astral) and they reincarnate on the physical plane without getting a taste of the fifth plane (mental). Lastly, the lowliest, mean, immoral persons, criminals, those living in pride, covetousness, lust, anger, gluttony, envy, sloth, etc., are expected to live for more than hundred years on the astral plane and they immediately reincarnate on earth without getting a glimpse of the heaven. These are the rough estimates; and there could be persons who would spend thousands of years on a subdivision of the astral plane before either reincarnating or proceeding to a higher plane. Similarly, there could be persons who would spend thousands of years in heaven before either reincarnating or proceeding to the causal plane. And then, there could be several higher souls who would proceed directly to the mental, intuitional or even the *atmic* plane, without spending a day on any of the lower planes. And again, there could be persons of the meanest and most heinous nature who may only live on the first subdivision of the astral plane for several thousands of years, before anything better or worse can happen to them.

The last words about mental plane. Like all other planes, this plane is also divided into seven subdivisions; the upper division, called the causal plane, is divided into three subdivisions, while the lower division, called the heaven, is subdivided into four subdivisions. Heaven is the giver of happiness unconditionally, since the astral body, which is the cause of desires, has already been dropped at the time of entry into the mental plane, which is after the second death. Life, in heaven, is self-contented since you do not need anything for living there. So much so that, even if you remember someone related to you on the physical plane, he appears before you in his real form, whether he is living on earth, is dead or has reincarnated.

2
THE SOUL OR *ATMAN*

Introduction

Sixth century B.C. is unforgettable since it saw the birth of "spiritual giants" around the world; Buddha and Mahavira in India, Pythagoras in Greece, Confucius in China, Zoroaster in Persia, and Druids in Europe, all made history on the path of Self-realisation. This was no ordinary event; either the "super human mind" beyond earth initiated it or, more rationally, the human evolution had reached the stage of spiritual quest. And after this, a series of persons kept on emerging on the spiritual path in all parts of the world. In the same way, the nineteenth century should be remembered for the birth of three geniuses who emphasised the existence of soul or *atman*; they were, Madame H.P. Blavatsky (1831-1891) of Russia, Sri Aurobindo Ghose (1872-1950) of India and Carl Gustav Jung (1875-1961) of Switzerland. Martinus (1890-1981) of Denmark got an independent realisation and presented his theory of soul and God. (Larsson 1963) It was at the same time that the turn of the present century saw the birth of "quantum physics", which tends to provide in a way, the scientific proof of the "existence of the soul or *atman*", in confirmation with the timeless "perennial philosophy" of the religions. It is found that the attributes of the soul are similar to the properties of the "electron", and hence the soul can be known and understood through the electron. It can be inferred that the soul is the non-local aspect of the human beings.

Sir Fred Hoyle, F.R.S., scientist and astronomer, questioned the basic propositions of scientific theory and he has subsequently established a reputation for brilliant and radical thought. (Lello 1985, 24) He has been associated with the "steady state theory of the universe" and has been developing the "meaning of existence" in the finest scientific tradition. He concluded that the Darwinian theory is wrong; it does not explain the crucial question of variations among the species. Sir Hoyle believes that the basic information we have has come from outside the earth. He believes that life did not start on earth, rather somewhere else. According to him, the Big Bang theory does not lead to a connection between the early stages and what we see now, and hence it is wrong. In his opinion, the religionist cannot understand the origin of man and so he thinks that man must have been created somehow, which is wrong. Similarly, the scientist's thinking that matter must have been created by the Big Bang because he cannot understand where matter came from, is also wrong. The universe, he feels, must have evolved from some previous conditions. The Big Bang is like trying to build a large building on quicksands, while the Steady State provides a firm backdrop against which events could work out. In other words, there is a guiding intelligence which has ordered something. He thinks that the intelligence in the universe is trying to cope with something but cannot give perfect solutions. We are, perhaps, a small reflection of the intelligence which produced us. One may say that we are the local representatives of the larger intelligence, and this, as he thinks, conforms to some extent to formal religions.

Professor Hoyle thinks that we may be heading towards the stage where the objective may not be too far. "The religious people have got it with St. Paul on the road to Damascus. The sudden light – it's just like that in science. There is a turning point." (Lello 1985, 31) Laboratory tests leading to the conclusion that the tiny particles in space have a very decisive property, was the moment on the road to Damascus for him. Particles in space have the characteristics of living material, which he calls the "infrared thumbprint". It is just a feeling within yourself, it is light on the road to Damascus. Sir Hoyle is impressed by the remarks of Einstein that "God may be subtle but He is not malicious," in which he seems to have summed up the whole scientific philosophy. Life possesses the universal thumbprint property and we are a component in a large-scale system. When enough people have gone through the crisis on the road to Damascus and form a sort of caucus opinion, they begin to teach this to others.

Sir Hoyle feels that the formal religion is a three-thousand-year-old prejudice; unless people can get away from this prejudice and from the scientist without a religion, another planet will have failed. Nevertheless, there are many planets and some get through, but the world is not in a good situation. In his own words, "We have reached the stage where we can destroy ourselves a hundred times over in half an hour and that is a pretty grim possibility. Unless people sort themselves out, I do not think there is much time ahead. Although many things that I've said are not favourable to religion in detail, this business of a religious instinct, the sanctity of truth and so on, are signposts that will prevent our self-destruction." (Lello 1985, 34) On January 13, 1998, I saw on Discovery Channel in Denmark, a programme named "Search for other intelligent being in universe" in which Dr. Paul Butler and Dr. Chris Burrows took part. An important observation made in that programme, was "...whenever someone is advanced enough to contact other planets like us, they invariably design a self-destruction system like the atom bomb. That is why we have not heard from anyone so far." I may further add here the predictions of Nostradamus, made some 400 years ago, according to which the world might see the end of civilisation in 1999. However, there is a possibility that the "saving programme" may already have started as Sir Hoyle has hinted earlier in this paragraph.

Sir Alister Hardy, F.R.S., commenting upon the term "road to Damascus" used frequently by Sir Fred Hoyle in *Revelations – Glimpses of Reality*, says that the term means a "sudden revelation", or something very important which influences the whole outlook of the individual, to which he might give the name of God. He further says, "I felt intellectually ashamed of the modern academic attitude to what one might call the study of the nature of life. The most important feature about living things is the nature of consciousness. At present, it is largely ignored, because one cannot see a method of investigating it; but there can be no doubt that it is there, and not just confined to man." (Lello 1985, xiv)

Although Blavatsky, Aurobindo, Jung and Martinus did not have the after-life or beyond-death in mind, their proposition of the spirit or soul fits completely well with the properties of the "astral plane" above earth and the other higher realms. The blending of the two – the scientific electron, and the religious soul and higher realms of various scriptures – tends to give a very good explanation of the "Creation" of God. The present chapter endeavours to prove the non-locality and general quantum nature of the soul, through this blending of the "psi-evidence", "quantum physics", the "experiences of the saints" and the "descriptions in various scriptures".

Twentieth century has produced a large number of spiritual giants in recent years, who have given a lucid and exhaustive explanation of soul and God in their writings. Notable amongst them are Ramakrishna Paramahansa, Vivekananda, Yukteswar (1984), Yogananda (1986), Meher Baba (1967), Muktananda (1972), Sivananda (1991), Gopi Krishna (1971), Vishnu Tirtha (1993), Asaramji (1994), Satyananda Saraswati (1984) and Vimalananda (Svoboda 1993). Anne Bancroft (1976) has given a brief survey of the saints of the present century in *Twentieth Century Mystics and Sages.*

Religion and Science

Religion existed long before science came into being; the latter being only about 500 years old, perhaps with the invent of astronomy by the pioneers, such as Galileo and Copernicus. Since science deals with objectivity, it appeals to the human mind easily as the scientific results can be seen through the eyes made of flesh. On the other hand, subjectivity of religion is not easy to grasp since one has to become a part of the process oneself and the results are only experienced subjectively, they cannot be shown objectively. It is at this stage that Descartes separated science from religion some 400 years ago. But now, at the so-called New Age, especially with the invent of quantum physics, the physicists are perhaps losing grip on reality, although they do not want to admit it publicly at present. (Herbert 1987, 15) Paul Twitchell of Eckankar said that religion and science are going to merge into each other and a new theory is going to emerge in the 21st century. J. B. Rhine also began to show the signs of fatigue in his later years when no physical or mathematical models could possibly be fitted into any of the paranormal phenomena being experimented at the Duke University. In fact, physicist Morris admitted that whatever concessions physics may give to paranormal phenomena, no explanation can ever be possible. (Morris and Edge 1986) I would go a step further and hypothesise that science is eventually going to lose its identity and finally merge into religion. More and more scientists are now admitting that they cannot explain phenomena until they become a part of it by way of meditation. And when this happens, religion and paranormal will remain, and science will vanish. The Discovery Channel on television has been giving programme in which well-known scientists have opined that it may never by possible to go beyond our own solar system because of two reasons: (i) the technology is extremely difficult, if not impossible, and (ii) when science has advanced to this stage, it has already developed a means of total destruction of the civilisation. This appears to be the reason why no one from space has been able to contact us on earth so far. To see that science has been following religion, by arriving at the conclusions long back held by religion, we proceed as follows.

Innumerable instances can be quoted from Hindu scriptures where the special character "Narad Muni" disappears at one place and instantly reappears at another place and communicates with another "being" instantly without opening his mouth. Time in *swarglok* (heaven on lower mental plane) moves extremely slowly for example, a person after spending about a year or so in *swarglok*, found on return to earth that two to three generations had passed there and his name and record could be found in some kind of an archive. Lord Krishna used to appear with a large number of *gopis* (milkmaids) simultaneously at several places, when they were involved in *ras lila* (a group dance). You could only spot a being on a higher realm, such as *swarglok*; there was no question of measuring one's speed since one could disappear and reappear instantly, from one place to another, irrespective of the distance between the two places.

Happenings described above are the normal characteristics of the astral and mental planes, discussed in Chapter 1. These are also experienced by yogis and saints from time to time on earth. Scientists, however, are only beginning to get a taste of such happenings through the study of an electron in quantum physics. Physicist Amit Goswami (1993, 9) has stated the following set of quantum properties:

i) A quantum object (for example, an electron) can be at more than one place at the same time (*the wave property*).
ii) A quantum object cannot be said to manifest in ordinary space-time reality until we observe it as a particle (*collapse of the wave*).
iii) A quantum object ceases to exist here and simultaneously appears in existence over there; we cannot say it went through the intervening space (*the quantum jump*).

iv) A manifestation of one quantum object, caused by our observation, simultaneously influences its correlated twin object – no matter how far apart they are (*quantum action-at-a-distance*).

My hypothesis is that the quantum properties described above become natural tools of a person on higher realms, the moment he discards the limited physical cover. And, of course, these properties become more and more refined as the person moves to a realm higher than the others. The behaviour of the subatomic particles on the physical plane is analogous to the behaviour of the people on higher realms, since the astral and higher bodies are subatomic in nature. To understand "soul" and to see that it has the above "quantum properties", we shall discuss them later in this chapter.

The *Secret Doctrine* of Blavatsky has the following conclusion: "Everything in the Universe, throughout all its kingdom, is conscious, i.e. endowed with a consciousness of its own kind and on its own plane of perception." (Blavatsky 1980-1988, 274) The torchbearer of Sri Aurobindo, Satprem of France, says, "The future belongs to those who give themselves unreservedly to the future. And we assert that there exists a future far more marvellous than all the electronic paradises of the mind: man is not the end... We seem to invent ever more marvellous machines, ceaselessly expand the limits of the human, even progress towards Jupiter and Venus. But that is only a seeming, increasingly deceptive and oppressive, and we do not expand anything. We merely send to the other end of the cosmos a pitiful little being who does not even know how to take care of his own kind, or whether his caves harbour a dragon or a mewling baby. We do not progress; we inordinately inflate an enormous mental balloon, which may well be exploding our face. We have not improved man; we have merely colossalised... The truth is, the summit of man – or the summit of anything at all – does not lie in perfecting to a higher degree the type under consideration; it lies in a 'something else' that is not of the same type and that he aspires to become. Such is the evolutionary law." (Satprem 1985, 4-5) And again, "The central point is the new understanding of the universe which is no longer perceived as consisting of solid bodies moving in space and time but rather, according to quantum theory, as a field of energy pervaded by consciousness. Western scientists, for the first time, have seriously faced the fact that if they want to understand the universe, they have to understand their own consciousness. A leader in this development was David Bohm, for he was one of the first scientists to take seriously the place of consciousness in scientific understanding." (Beversluis 1995, 282)

Above paragraph emphasises only one point, that "the scientific achievements, which are of the very finite nature, may be good for the physical comforts of the humans, and they may continue; however, to understand the infinite universe, one has to concentrate on the consciousness". What the universe is, has already been defined in Chapter 1. And what the consciousness is, it is the understanding of the infinite potentialities which we already possess; the sample of which has been demonstrated by the quantum electron; and the understanding of the universe through it.

I now proceed to answer the questions posed by Claire Walker, "Does consciousness work on the principle of non-locality? Are souls non-local and also psychic? If soul is psyche, then is the soul non-local aspect of a human being?" (Walker 1997, 135) The answer to all these questions is in the affirmative. To see this, we proceed as follows:

Subliminal of Sri Aurobindo and Collective Unconscious of Jung

The two great contemporary thinkers, independent of each other and treading divergent paths, converging at the same conclusion – that behind the conscious mind of the individual lies the unlimited psychic region, which constitutes as real a world as the physical one – was no ordinary event; perhaps, it was one of the most outstanding achievements of the present century. Although the facts have been known to various religions in varying degree for a long time, the present world needs some logic and some kind of proof before one can believe the mysticism found in religions, and this has been very well provided by these two giants of the present era. Subjectivity has been converted into "objective study" and "direct experiences". Jung arrived at his conclusions which were based on his own dreams and the dreams of his patients, while Sri Aurobindo's conclusions were based on his direct experiences through yoga and meditation. However, during his visions of death in 1944, Jung also had direct experiences in which he found himself floating "in a state of purest bliss thronged around with images of all creation", and the physical world appeared to him "downright ridiculous" and as a "segment of existence which is enacted in a three-dimensional box-like universe especially set up for it." (Jung 1961, 274-275) In his own words, "I would never have imagined that any such experience was possible. It was not a product of imagination. The visions and experience were utterly real; there was nothing subjective about them; they all had a quality of absolute objectivity... We shy away from the word 'eternal', but I can describe the experience only as the ecstasy of a non-temporal state in which present, past and future are one." (Jung 1961,

275) Nevertheless, his scientific way of writing, developed methodically, forced him to explain the supra-physical also in terms of the physical. "He could not discriminate between different ingredients of visions and archetypes. This has resulted in a lot of confusion in his theory of archetypes." (Singh 1986, 73)

There is an obscure region below the conscious mind which is called "unconscious" by Jung, and he divided it in two parts – personal and collective. The unconscious of Jung is the "subconscient" of Sri Aurobindo, who divided it in two parts – individual and universal – analogous to the divisions by Jung. Personal unconscious or individual subconscient is the storehouse of "suppressed and subsided material" from the present life, which was once floating in the conscious mind. "This material remains in the seed form in the subconscient and comes up again when it can." (Sri Aurobindo 1970, 357) Dreams in the sleeping state are nothing but the unfoldment of these impressions. Universal subconscient, on the other hand, comes from the inconscient, which is also the source of the conscious mind of the man, and of the instincts and impulses for life. Universal subconscient or the collective unconscious is formed in the process of evolution, right from the plant life and the animal kingdom, and it is the heritage of man. Both thinkers agree that this stratum of psyche is autonomous; and they attribute to it direct and immediate knowledge of objects and events. It preserves the past and reflects to it direct and immediate knowledge of objects and events. It preserves the past and reflects the future, for example, dreams predicting future events. According to both of them, it is the immeasurable sea from which the conscious mind has emerged simply as an iceberg. It is the source of paranormal phenomena, such as telepathy, telekinesis, clairvoyance, etc. Ordinarily, this part of the psyche is unapproachable to the conscious mind; it is only in the abnormal states or dreams that it reveals itself.

According to Sri Aurobindo, the universal subconscient, which is of the evolutionary origin, is only the lower part of the subliminal. The higher subliminal is due to the direct descent of the superconscient to the principle of mind, life and matter. According to both authors, the conscious mind receives the knowledge of its future course through the intuitions of the collective unconscious, and this cannot be the mere history of the conscious. According to Sri Aurobindo, higher subliminal is a part of the *atman* and "it is that which endures and is imperishable in us from birth to birth, untouched by death, decay or corruption, an indestructible spark of the Divine". (Sri Aurobindo 1970, 268-269) It is through *sadhana* that a yogi passes through the lower regions, encounters personal memories which block his inner growth and, finally, the subliminal consciousness expands into the "cosmic consciousness". (Aurobindo 1970, 644) "Just as Freud, in his idea of the unconscious, had confused the personal unconscious and the collective unconscious which, as Jung has shown, are entirely of different origin and nature, so Jung, in his idea of the collective unconscious, seems to have confused the lower and the higher spheres of the subliminal which, as shown by Sri Aurobindo, are still more disparate from each other in their origin and nature." (Singh 1986, 42)

The "archetype" of Jung is the "visionary being" of Sri Aurobindo. Noumenon of Kant seeks to express itself through the phenomenon; libido of Jung seeks to express itself through the consciousness; while the visions of Sri Aurobindo are considered by him as the Superconscious manifesting Itself in the form of Mind, Life and Matter.

Thus, the visions of Sri Aurobindo involve actual entities while the archetypes of Jung (including his anima and animus) are only forms or modes, not any particular character, in which the libido wants to express itself in a particular situation.

Sri Aurobindo divided visions into three distinct classes: the subtle physical, the vital and the mental. The first class deals with subtle causal form in which the awaiting future events of the universal nature are revealed. These events concern the gross physical world visible to the external eyes. The second class deals with the *intermediate zone* which concerns the beings of the vital world. These beings appear in different forms, including those of gods and goddesses or demons, and create problems for the practitioner, which he is supposed to transcend in order to proceed further on the spiritual path. These beings, in fact, may be called teachers or guides. The third class deals with the mental world, to which the practitioner qualifies after he has transcended the physical and vital worlds. As a result of mediation, the beings of mental plane appear as gods and goddesses of the *Vedas*, in the vision. These visions are actual manifestation in any of the lower worlds. Manifestation of the *Mother* is considered by Sri Aurobindo as the emanation from the Consciousness-Force (kinetic form of God or *Shakti*), which is the primary source of creation. The Mother can manifest on any of the lower planes. Likewise, *Satchidananda* (potential form of God or Shiva) is Lord Krishna of Sri Aurobindo, who also embodied the historical Krishna on earth – still living on a higher plane in the same form. The Mother or Lord Krishna can be contacted by the practitioner; he can see them and talk to them on the appropriate inner plane of higher consciousness. Various saints have had such experiences. I have described my own experiences earlier. (Kumar 1994)

The above three classes of visions are also talked of by Jung in the form of the future element of visions, Jungian gods and demons, and the Jungian archetypes of mother and Mandala. Sri Aurobindo got confirmation of his visions in yogic practices through myths and scriptures, and he was left with no doubts about their reality. On the other hand, Jung drew inferences from dreams and psychotic fantasies; and he could not change his mode of writing to which he got committed, although he himself had real visions in later life, as mentioned earlier.

Jung defined "ego" to be the result of "the collision between the somatic factor and the environment; it goes on developing from further collisions with the outer world and the inner". (Jung 1961, 5) Ego is the centre of the mental consciousness. It has its roots both in the "conscious personality" and in the "inner being". Its two divisions are called "manifest" and "unconscious substratum" by Jung, and "particular ego-sense" and "general ego-sense" by Sri Aurobindo. It thus represents the concentricity of both the inner and the outer being. Ego is very essential for the functioning of the sense organs, and hence for the action of the individual and one's adjustment to the environment. At the same time, it is the ego which is the source of all troubles in the humans, making them do inhuman acts. A representative becoming the master, it is like an anchor necessary to hold the ship near the shore for some time; and then, it should be released for the free movement of the ship. As another example, earth may be erroneously said to be the centre of the universe. The ignorance must be encountered, the anchor must be removed, the proper centre must be found and the ego must be replaced. Ego is not monolithic, it is both subjective and objective with respect to its own knowledge, and thus suffers with its proneness to the divisibility of the personality into these two disparate elements, as is obvious from the phenomenon of dream. Accordingly, ego cannot be the centre of the conscious being, and more so of the whole psyche, which is so vast and varied in its contents. Thus, there should be some other principle in the individual which is responsible for the unification of the disparate elements of the personality into a whole.

Sin and suffering are caused by the erroneous thinking by a person that he is the doer of an act, and thereby taking the onus on himself. He may wrongly think that he is carrying the bag in a flight from London to New York; while, in fact, it is the aeroplane which is carrying the bag from station A to station B. Someone out of employment may accuse a single person for his unemployment; but, if a careful analysis is carried out, it would be found that there are several reasons interwoven into each other, that no single factor can be held responsible for his being without job. Similarly, any particular act on earth is the result of the whole machinery, and not any single factor. "There is no such thing as chance." (Field 1976, 82) Things are happening by themselves; we wrongly think that we are the cause of a particular happening; and by doing so "sin" and "suffering" are invented unnecessarily. This is one of the most important teachings of the *Bhagavad Gita,* and one who has assimilated this wisdom in oneself is a liberated person. "The sense, the idea, the experience that I am separately self-existent being in the universe, and the forming of consciousness and force of being into the mould of that experience are the root of all suffering, ignorance and evil. And it is so because that falsifies both in practice and cognition the whole real truth of things; it limits the being, limits the consciousness, limits the power of our being, limits the bliss of being; this limitation, again produces a wrong way of existence, wrong way of consciousness, wrong way of using the power of our being and consciousness, and wrong, perverse and contrary forms of the delight of existence." (Sri Aurobindo n.d. 2, 779)

In Chapter 1, we saw the division of the universe into seven planes. Sri Aurobindo described the planes of human consciousness from downside upwards as follows: physical or material, vital, mental, subliminal and spiritual – which is fully congruent with the lower five planes talked of in the previous chapter. According to him, the human consciousness is composed of all the five states of consciousness put together, which is again in full agreement with the description in the mentioned chapter. As the person advances to higher levels, the lower levels of consciousness are automatically eliminated from one's composition. He called the group of "physical, vital and mental" consciousness as the *outer consciousness,* which concerns the environment around the individual. The group of higher levels of consciousness – higher mind, illumined mind, intuition and overmind, from lowest level upwards, which the individual is normally not aware of – was called by him as *inner or subliminal consciousness,* which is of the universal nature and which co-exists with Matter, Life and Mind. (Sri Aurobindo n.d. 3, 311-312) Thus, according to him too, the universe has seven levels of existence. It is the inner consciousness which is responsible for the dreams, visions and all kinds of paranormal faculties including the solution of otherwise unsolvable problems. The characteristic of an illumined mind is "simultaneity of comprehension", that of intuition is "abrupt illumination", and that of overmind is the "steady state of intuitive knowledge". At the fall of the wall between the outer and inner consciousness, a new consciousness dawns in the practitioner, called the *cosmic consciousness.* The individual "becomes directly aware of a universal being, universal state, universal force and power, universal Mind, Life, Matter and lives in constant relations with these things". (Sri Aurobindo 1958, part III, 1070) Dr. Richard Maurice Bucke has presented a detailed account of the lives and achievements of persons who were endowed with cosmic consciousness. (Bucke 1961) However, there are persons who achieved a consciousness higher than the cosmic, among the subjects described by Bucke, but he has not made any distinction of them from others.

Cosmic consciousness still suffers with its entanglement with the affairs of Nature. A state higher than the cosmic, which is characterised with the oneness and freedom of the Absolute-*Satchidananda*, is called *spiritual or supramental consciousness* by Sri Aurobindo. In this state, the subject and object become one, or in other words, the "seer, seeing and seen" become one. "We enter into the awareness of self, the Spirit, the Divine, and are able to see in all things their essential reality and the play of forces and phenomena as preceding from that essential reality." (Sri Aurobindo 1958, 316)

There is a "conscious personality" representing the "inner world", having a sense of wholeness and unity of both the conscious and unconscious minds; unlike the ego which unifies only the conscious mind, it must be a greater principle than ego; it is this conscious personality which is called the "supra-ordinate personality" and given the name of "Self" by Jung. Thus, ego is only a derivative of the Self and it is related to the Self as the object to the subject.

Both Jung and Sri Aurobindo found the real centre to be the "Self", which has the unitary nature and represents the inner reality in its totality. Both of them found that the Self is indivisible and because of it being the complete representative of the psyche, it was regarded to be omnipresent. According to Jung, it is the common centre of both the conscious and the unconscious. Sri Aurobindo considers it to be the original centre of pure consciousness, and a finite representative of the infinite. In his view, it is the real "I", *Atman,* the Highest *Purusha,* "secret soul" or Self; transcendent (combining diversity and unity, and individual and universal) and eternal; at once wheel and motion, centre and circumference. (Aurobindo 1970, 660) It can both be inferred logically and realised in meditation, "extending itself upward into a transcendence of which the limits are not visible". (Aurobindo 1970, 108) According to Jung, "Under certain conditions the unconscious spontaneously brings forth an archetypal symbol of wholeness." (Jung 1961, 69) Referring to India's theory of *atman,* which unifies the complementary elements of consciousness and the unconscious, he said, *atman* "on the one hand embraces the universe and on the other is 'not bigger than a thumb' dwelling in the heart". (Jung 1961, Vol. XIV, 122) Jung observed that the man first disclaimed the Self due to the arrogance of the ego and now he is desperate in his search of the same. Yet, however, one must keep a balance between the ego and the Self for everything to go well, in accordance with the law of opposites, which states that everything requires for its existence its own opposite, or else it fades into nothingness. "It is only separation, detachment and agonising confrontation through opposition that produce consciousness and insight." (Jung 1961, Vol. IX, Part I, 171)

When we talk about God, perhaps, we are touching the most important part of our discussion. In several religions, including Christianity, Hinduism and Sufism, the "archetype of Self" has been called God. According to Jung, "Christ, who is a typical manifestation of the Self, is regarded as the central figure in the Divine Trinity. In Hinduism, it is represented by *Atman* which is regarded as identical with *Brahman*." (Jung 1961, Vol. V, 391-393) According to Sri Sankaracharya, "*Brahman* and *Atman* which are designated by the terms 'that' and 'thou', respectively, are fully proved to be identical when investigated by the light of Vedic teaching." (Chatterji 1932, 94) In the words of Aldous Huxley, "Based upon the direct experience of those who have fulfilled the necessary conditions of such knowledge, this teaching is expressed most succinctly in the Sanskrit formula, *tat tvam asi* (that thou art); the *Atman*, or imminent eternal Self, is one with Brahman, the Absolute Principle of all existence; and the last end of every human being is to discover the fact for himself, to find out who he really is." (Huxley 1944, 1-2) Merwan Sheriar Irani, a Sufi Muslim saint of this century, popularly known as Meher Baba, said that human psyche has two parts, one part falls within the range of consciousness and the other part falls beyond it. "The unconscious part, in its full extent, is identical with the power which is behind matter. It is referred to as God by the orthodox religions. The Ultimate Reality which is symbolically represented through such concepts can be known fully only by bringing the unconscious into conscious." (Baba 1967, Vol. II, 39)

Sri Aurobindo calls the Ultimate Reality as *Satchidananda*; that is, *sat* (existence), *chit* (consciousness) and *ananda* (bliss). The creative power of *Satchidananda* is called by him as Consciousness-Force. Thus "consciousness" is the inherent nature of God and His creative energy. Psychologically, neither Jung nor Sri Aurobindo could conclude whether it was consciousness or the unconscious, which came first into existence. Sri Aurobindo then took refuge with metaphysics and declared that *Satchidananda* goes into self-concealment Himself for evolution to take place. The highest stage of evolution is man, the level at which unconsciousness is thrown completely in the background and consciousness becomes all-prominent. The moment unconscious is brought into conscious, Self-realisation, and hence, God-realisation takes place. Sri Aurobindo describes Self-realisation in these words, "The status or action in us of an inherent, intrinsic, self-existent consciousness which knows itself by the mere fact of being, knows all that is in itself in the same way, by identity with it, begins even to see all that to our mind seems external in the same manner, by a movement of identity or by an intrinsic direct consciousness which envelopes, penetrates, enters into its object, discovers itself in the object, is aware in it of something in it of something that is not mind or life or body." (Sri Aurobindo 1970, 1019)

Experiences of Sri Aurobindo

In the words of Sri Aurobindo (on retiring in a room for three days with a yogi in 1907, and meditating), "The first result was a series of tremendously powerful experiences and radical changes of consciousness which I had never intended and which were quite contrary to my own ideas, for they made me see with a stupendous intensity the world as a cinematographic play of vacant forms in the impersonal universality of the Absolute Brahman... It threw me suddenly into a condition above and without thought, unstained by any mental or vital movement; there was no ego, no real world... This was no mental realisation, nor something glimpsed somewhere above, no abstraction; it was positive, the only positive reality... What it brought was an expressible Peace, a stupendous silence, an infinity of release and freedom. (While confined to a solitary cell in jail for one month in 1908) I looked at the jail that secluded me from men and it was no longer by its high walls that I was prisoned; no, it was Vasudeva who surrounded me. I walked under the branches of the tree in front of my cell but it was not the tree, I knew it was Vasudeva, it was Sri Krishna whom I saw standing there and holding over me his shade. I looked at the bars of my cell, the very grating that did duty for a door and again I saw Vasudeva. It was Narayana who was guarding and sending sentry over me. Or I lay on the coarse blankets that were given me for a couch and I felt the arms of Sri Krishna around me, the arms of my friend and lover... I looked at the prisoners in the jail, the thieves, the murderers, the swindlers, and as I looked at them, I saw Vasudeva, it was Narayana whom I found in these darkened souls and misused bodies." (Satprem n.d. 157-169)

In the words of the host of Sri Aurobindo, "One felt when he spoke as if somebody else was speaking through him. I placed the plate of food before him, he simply gazed at it, then ate a little, just mechanically. He appeared to be absorbed even when he was eating; he used to meditate with open eyes... Without falling into ecstatic trance, with eyes wide open, Sri Aurobindo found himself precipitated into the Supreme Light." (Satprem n.d. 268-269)

Sri Aurobindo fasted, slept very little, experimented with the principles of spiritual life very methodically, and finally put them into writing. In his own words, "I have been testing day and night, for years upon years, more scrupulously than any scientist his theory or his method on the physical plane." (Satprem n.d., 331)

He was mentally subjected to all sorts of torture for fifteen days and he had to look upon pictures of all sorts of suffering, before the final transformation of the consciousness took place. From 1910 to 1950, his life was devoted to confirmation, expansion, consolidation and practical application of the spiritual experiences gained by him. In 1920, Madame Mirra Richard of France was entrusted with the charge of the *Ashram* in Pondicherry. Also, having considered his writings as sufficient, he discontinued the journal *Arya*. Freeing himself from all the tasks in this way, he then devoted himself to the practice of yoga more intensively. He attained complete *siddhi* on November 24, 1926. Afterwards, he withdrew himself completely into seclusion; only the Mother and a few selected people could see him. He left his physical body on December 5, 1950.

Experiences of Carl Jung

"Of course, in Jung also, particularly in his later experiences, we find a certain circumspection in this regard which throws him unmistakably into the arms of spirituality. In the visions of death which he had in 1944, he felt himself floating 'in a state of purest bliss thronged round with images of all creation'. In contrast to the world of inner states, the physical world appeared to him as 'downright ridiculous'. He viewed this life as a 'segment of existence which is enacted in a three-dimensional box-like universe especially set up for it'. He himself was stunned by the surprising objectivity of the world of visions." (Singh 1986, 72) In the words of Jung himself, "I would never have imagined that any such experience was possible. It was not a product of imagination. The visions and experience were utterly real; there was nothing subjective about them; they all had a quality of absolute objectivity... We shy away from the word 'eternal', but I can describe the experience only as the ecstasy of a non-temporal state in which present, past and future are one." (Jung 1961, 275)

Jung was well conversant with yoga and meditation also, as one can see from his following dream, "I was on a hiking trip. I was walking along a little road through a hilly landscape; the sun was shining and I had a wide view in all directions. Then I came to a small way-side chapel. The door was ajar and I went in. To my surprise, there was no image of the Virgin on the altar, and no crucifix either, but only a wonderful flower arrangement. But then I saw that on the floor in front of the altar, facing me, sat a yogi in lotus posture, in deep meditation. When I looked at him closely, I realised that he had my face. I started in profound fright, and awoke with the thought, 'Aha, so he is the one who is meditating on me. He has a dream, and I am it.'" (Jung 1961, 299) "Jung treats this dream as a parable and understands himself, the dreamer as the ego, and the *yogi* as the self. According to him, assumption of the human form by the self is indicative of its entering into the three-dimensional existence. The thought arising immediately after the dream is taken to reflect the relationship between the self and the ego, the latter being treated as meditation within the former along with the apprehension that the ego would evaporate into nothingness as soon as the meditation would come to an end." (Singh 1986, 84-85)

Experiences of Savitri

When Savitri turns inward in search of the soul, the last part of the journey in the spiritual consciousness, where she realises the Self ultimately, has the following account, (Sri Aurobindo n.d. 3, 594-595)

> In the last chamber on a golden seat
> One sat whose shape no vision could define,
> Only one felt the world's unattainable fount,
> A power of which she was a straying Force,
> An invisible Beauty, goal of the world's desire,
> A Sun of which all knowledge is beam,
> A Greatness without whom no life could be.
> Thence all departed in silent self,
> And all became formless and pure and bare.
> Then through a tunnel dug in the last rock
> She came out where there shone a deathless sun,
> A house was there all made of flame and light
> And crossing a wall of doorless living fire
> There suddenly she met her secret soul.

Experiences of William Wordsworth

Realisation of the Self (Soul) by William Wordsworth is obvious from the following passage from his book *Intimations of Immortality*, (Zemke 1996, 156)

> Our birth is but a sleep and a forgetting;
> The soul that rises with us, our life star,
> Hath had elsewhere, its setting,
> And cometh from afar.
> Not in entire forgetfulness,
> And not in utter nakedness,
> But trailing clouds of glory do we come
> From God, who is our home.

Experiences of Saint Asaramaji (1994)

"*Paramatma* is the source of cosmic energy which activates our consciousness. That consciousness makes the world of dreams in *Hita* nerve. That consciousness in paralytic state is converted into deep sleep. Attainment of *Atma-Paramatma,* awareness or knowledge of It for a period of even three minutes by someone will not let one suffer the agony of being in the womb of a mother again. One becomes a liberated soul."

To understand the reality of the "soul", we move on.

The Horizontal and the Vertical

The horizontal aspect of living is concerned with life as a physical being in a material world, where, indeed, development at an acceptable level is an essential of satisfying life. (Walker 1997, 75) Establishment of one's identity, development of meaningful connections with others, achievement of a certain level of security and recognition – enough for the continuation of one's development, is a necessary first step. (See, for example, Zukav 1989) Dr. Annie Besant finds it natural to play with the *toys* – pleasure, money, power, honour; for satisfaction and for the development of the human will, mental power and emotional strength; and, when the toys break, it opens the way for the expansion of the higher faculties and values. (Besant 1923, 213) The transition from horizontal to vertical aspiration takes place when the psychic needs of everyday living are in balance, and an individual feels secure enough, free enough to give attention to a new set of values. (Walker 1997, 77) Jiddu Krishnamurti repeatedly asserted in his lectures that an inner order is a prerequisite to an outward order, and this is what I have tried to bring out in my paper "Psychic Individuation and Self-Realisation" with respect to the relationship between men and women. (Kumar 1997, July)

The totality of psychological principles, fields and functions in an individual is defined as *psyche* by Jung. According to him, "The lower reaches of the psyche begin where the function emancipates itself from the impulsive forces of 'instinct' and becomes amenable to the will." This is in agreement with the point elaborated in the above paragraph. Psyche has two parts – conscious and unconscious. "The subjectivity of the conscious psyche lies in its being subject to the operation of the ego, while the objectivity of the unconscious pscyhe consists in its being autonomous." (Jung n.d. 1, Vol. XII, 43-45) Although conscious and unconscious are supposed to be exclusive to each other, he did not rule out the possibility of the fact that "there is no unconscious psychism which is not at the same time conscious." (Jung n.d. 1, Vol. XII, 200) Accordingly, one has to consider both the conscious and the unconscious simultaneously, without giving priority to one over the other, if we have to understand the psyche in a full way. "To these are to be added *the ego and the self as centres of the conscious and unconscious respectively.*" (Jung n.d. 1, Vol. VIII, 151-152) This suggests that the horizontal is represented by the conscious ego while the vertical is represented by the unconscious self.

Psyche is Universal, Collective, Eternal, Unique, a Cosmic Principle and Existence Itself.

Although constituted of the disparate elements, psyche functions as a whole. During sleep, consciousness disappears, yet we remember dreams. This, together with the paranormal phenomena – telepathy, telekinesis, precognition, levitation, etc. – experimented at the Duke

University and other centres, shows the universality of the psyche. It has the whole history of the organic evolution due to the principle of hereditary transmission; this shows its collectiveness. Because of its non-spatial and non-temporal character, Jung regards pscyhe to be eternal and describes it to be "*a mathematical point and at the same time as a universe of fixed stars*". (Jung n.d. 1, Vol. VIII, 414, 348) Because of it being a source of consciousness, Jung calls it a "cosmic principle", and because of its trans-spatial, trans-temporal and accusal properties, he regards it to be "unique" in itself and probably capable of constituting another dimension of the universe, besides the temporal and the spatial. (Jung n.d. 1, 282-283). Because of all these properties, Jung regards the psyche to be a miniature universe in itself. The inter-dependence of psyche and matter is obvious from his following statement, "Psyche cannot be totally different from matter, for how otherwise could it move matter? And matter cannot be alien to psyche, for how otherwise could it move matter? And matter cannot be alien to psyche, for how else could matter produce psyche? Psyche and matter exist in one and the same world, and each partakes of the other, otherwise any reciprocal action would be impossible." (Jung n.d. 1, Vol. IX, Part II, 261). "In fact, Jung regards psyche and matter as co-ordinate entities, each constituting the pre-condition of the existence of the other. If psyche without brain is inconceivable, the external world without consciousness is a virtual non-entity. Hence, Jung characterises the psyche not only as existent but also as 'existence itself'." (Singh 1986, 118)

We thus find two virtually opposing contents in psyche – matter and spirit. They give rise to animals or subhuman entities as a requirement of instincts and biological needs on one hand, and to archetypal divine entities for the satisfaction of the spiritual needs on the other. The pull of the two against each other creates friction and generates "psychic energy", called "libido" by Jung. Freud was the first to use the word libido as the "sexual drive" creating energy for all psychological purposes. Jung called libido a general life instinct originating from the Sanskrit word *lobha*. According to him, it is "an energy valve which is able to communicate itself to any field of activity whatever, be it power, hunger, hatred, sexuality or religion, without ever being itself a specific instinct". (Jung n.d. 1, Vol. V, 136-137) Jung compared psychic energy to physical energy and tried to govern it by the formula given by Einstein, with the difference that physical energy is related to quantity of mass while psychic energy is related to quality of spiritual force. "As we rise higher in the psychic sphere, the hold of instincts goes on lessening gradually, until at last the psyche achieves complete autonomy and 'attains a so-called spiritual form'." (Jung n.d. 1, Vol. VIII, 181)

Jung divides the personality in two parts, inner and outer, which are in counterbalance with each other. The inner personality, which includes the inner attitude, the character, that is turned towards the unconscious, is the manner of one's behaviour towards the inner psychic processes. The outer one is called by him as "persona", while the inner one is called as anima/animus or "soul". (Jung n.d. 2, 593) His way of defining soul differs from the traditional Christian way. However, it is the *psyche* which he defines to be "the totality of all the psychic processes, both conscious as well as unconscious". (Jung n.d. 2, 588) *Thus, it is the "psyche" which corresponds to the traditional definition of "soul" in various religions and to the "atman" of the Hindus.* According to him, *Atman* is the one which "on the one hand embraces the universe and on the other is 'not bigger than a thumb' dwelling in the heart." (Jung 1961, Vol. XIV, 122)

The co-existence of things may be taken as the *horizontal* part of the world, while the intensity and tangibility of things can be regarded as the *vertical* part of it. Thus, something that appears to be out of place may be the index of some universal activity. Both Jung and Sri Aurobindo admit the *existence of the worlds beyond the physical.* On "the hypothetical possibility that the psyche touches on a form of existence outside space and time", and the validity of this possibility through the "relativisation of the space category by the modern theoretical physics", Jung is inclined to believe the existence beyond space, time and the law of causality. (Jung n.d. 1, Vol. VIII, 414) Sri Aurobindo divides the existence into two parts: one, concentric or outer, and the other, vertical or inner. Outer rings are made of "our ordinary exterior mind, life, body consciousness", while the inner rings are made of "an inner mind, an inner life, an inner physical consciousness". (Sri Aurobindo 1958, Part I, 251) The inner mind preserves the entire history of evolution in condensed form and sees the future as clearly as it sees the present, unlike the outer mind which depends on approximation through inference. It is also the source of predictive dreams. Sri Aurobindo believed in the co-existence of *horizontal and vertical lives,* and hence on the existence of a world of mind, a world of life along with the world of matter, based on the law of continuity in nature. He calls the "psychic existence" of the group of inner vital and inner physical forms by the name *subliminal,* of which a person is normally unaware. The subliminal is vindicated for its vast consciousness through dreams and yogic experiences, and through abnormal states of mind which provide solutions to problems otherwise not easy to solve.

Sri Aurobindo views "ego" to be the centre of the surface mind and "psychic being" to be the centre of the subliminal, located just behind the heart, unlike emotions which emanate from the front part of the heart. (Sri Aurobindo n.d. 2, 206-207) The psychic being is also called the "Purusha in the heart" or "Chaitya Purusha". Referring to *Sat-Chit-Ananda,* it has originated from the third cosmic principle *Ananda,* "the delight-soul in the universe". (Sri Aurobindo n.d. 2, 843) Although it is the centre of the subliminal, it lies beyond the inner mental, inner vital and inner physical; and, it is the permanent referee of these three forms. It has "a direct touch upon truth" and one meets it as the *profounder mystic light* at the fourth centre of energy, called the *anahat chakra.* (Sri Aurobindo n.d. 2, 170) *Jivatman, atman,* or "soul" is an eternal fraction of the Divine and it dwells always in the knowledge or self-awareness of *Satchidananda.* At the initial stages of involution of *Satchidananda*, the soul remains dormant; however, when it asserts itself, an individuality evolves from within the soul and is manifested as the "psychic being". Thus, it is "the soul-form or soul-personality developed through this evolution". (Sri Aurobindo 1958, 341) It grows as the personality of the soul, controls all the factors of the subliminal, and serves as the "central being in the evolution". (Sri Aurobindo 1958, 279) As a direct representative of *atman,* it has all the knowledge of the universal reality inherent in it, and gradually, it tends to become omniscient.

The Self is the centre of our being in totality which continues from birth to birth and which supervises and supports us for everything. It manifests itself in two forms

– *jivatman* and psychic being. "While the *jivatman* remains unaffected by birth and death, the psychic being is quite involved in them. While the *jivatman*, as a portion of the Divine, is universal as well as individual, the psychic being narrows itself down to sheer individuality... It, indeed, is the carrier of the experiences from life to life. According to Sri Aurobindo, as well as the *Upanishads*, there is a personal formation on each plane of our being, the physical, the vital, the mental and the supramental. These formations are known as *Purushas*. Thus, there is a physical, a vital, a mental and a psychic *Purusha*, each forming the centre of its own plane. "When the soul or spark of the Divine Fire" begins to develop a psychic individuality, observes Sri Aurobindo, "that psychic individuality is called the psychic being". "When the psychic being gains dominance over the mental, the vital and the physical, it makes use of them as its instruments. This is described by Sri Aurobindo as psychic transformation." (Singh 1986, 133-134)

Remarks

Before proceeding further to the individuation of Jung and transformation of Sri Aurobindo, which leads to the theory of *kundalini* in the next chapter, I would like to halt here to evince the psychic properties of the soul. The "psyche" of Jung or the *atman* of Sri Aurobindo is seen to be universal, collective, eternal, unique, a cosmic principle and existence itself. It is the "soul" of all the orthodox religions and is described as having the above properties by various scriptures. Details of the universe presented in Chapter 1 further suggest that the soul has all the paranormal properties, such as telepathy, clairvoyance, telekinesis, levitation, etc. There are various biographies and autobiographies which evince the above properties of the soul. For example, Paul Twitchell, the former spiritual head of Eckankar, could come out of his body at will and exhibit some of the above properties; see for details *In My Soul I Am Free* by Brad Steiger (n.d.). Some of these properties are found to be possessed by the quantum electron as stated by physicist Amit Goswami: the wave property, collapse of the wave, the quantum jump and quantum action-at-a-distance. (Goswami 1993, 9) According to these properties, an object can be at more than one place at the same time, it can manifest only when observed as a particle, it may cease to exist at one place and simultaneously appear at another place without going through the intervening space, and the manifestation of an object can influence its correlated twin object, no matter how far apart they are.

Two quantum properties – the Heisenberg's uncertainty principle and the principle of non-locality – are also found to be possessed by the souls. The first principle means that either the location or the speed of a quantum object can be measured at one time, not both. The second principle means that one body can influence the other, whatever distance they may have between them, and without an apparent exchange of force or energy between them.

True-life happenings are taking place round the world from time immemorial which suggest that the soul possesses all the above properties. Accordingly, I hypothesise that soul is not only non-local and quantum in its full content, but is has a large number of properties which are yet to be proved by quantum physics. I present some of the true-life cases from India in the following paragraphs. The authors of these writings, which have appeared in the Hindi magazine *Manohar Kahanian*, are still alive at the time of writing of this book and they can be easily contacted for verification.

True Life Cases Illustrating the Powers of the Soul

Case I

An assistant professor in the department of ancient history at the University of Delhi, accompanied Mr. Samarendra Singh and his sixteen-year-old daughter, Sarita, for the study of an old statue of an ancestor of Mr. Singh. The statue was situated in the backyard of an old palatial building, a few miles from the city of Benares in northern India.

The professor was stunned to see the statue. Although the statue was that of an Indian fighter, yet it carried an impression of medieval Italy. He had not seen such a beautiful and all-round, almost-perfect statue for a long time. Sarita was looking at it with wide open eyes. She simply whispered, "Marvellous." The statue had strings round the legs in Roman style, holding the sword with the right hand and its case with the left hand, wearing a pointed turban and moustaches, having big and impressive eyes, and it appeared as if he was just going to attack the enemy. Mr. Singh told Sarita that the statue belonged to one of their ancestors but he could not recollect the name. Sarita was looking at the statue with great admiration and respect and said, "How brave and attractive were our ancestors. I will never get tired looking at him." She bent her head very respectfully to salute the statue and she touched its feet with her hands. The professor and Mr. Singh were surprised to see this. She advised them as if they were small children and she was an elderly person, "Papa, he is our ancestor. It is our duty to pay respect to him." The two elders were ashamed to hear this and they too touched the feet of the statue with their hands.

The statue was a rare one and the professor and Mr. Singh were thinking about how to protect it form dacoits. The professor wanted to study it in detail, publish his work at the university, and suggested that it should be transferred to the museum in Delhi. In the meanwhile, the housekeeper Raghu, came and told them that the infamous dacoit Madho Singh was very active in that area in those days. Mr. Singh asked Raghu if the matter has been reported to the police or not. Raghu smiled sarcastically and told them that the group of the dacoit Madho Singh was so strong that even the police were afraid of them. Mr. Singh then said that it was his responsibility to look after the safety of the area and he would have to do something about it.

The same night, dacoit Madho Singh appeared in the area and entered the room of Mr. Singh with about ten heavily armed people. He was more than six feet tall and he had an athletic body. He picked up Sarita and carried her with him, all others were tied down with ropes. He told Mr. Singh that he should arrange for fifteen hundred thousand rupees within ten days from now, if he wanted his daughter back, otherwise she would be cut into four pieces and brought back here.

Everyone was upset, and was thinking about the future. Right at that time, there was a sound in the backyard, as if someone treading with very heavy feet. That sound moved backward and disappeared.

The nephew of Raghu opened the door of the room. He looked quite upset. He had come from the village. He informed the others that the dacoits had looted the people and they would now be going to the jungle of Bathia, some two miles behind the building they were staying in. Suddenly, someone shouted from the back of the house and everyone ran there. It was found that the statue had disappeared from its place. Everybody presumed that the dacoit Madho Singh had taken the statue also along with Sarita. They also speculated that the dacoits would sell it to a big smuggler for several hundred thousand rupees. Everyone, especially Mr. Singh, was thinking about the miserable condition in which his daughter Sarita may by living under the control of the torturous dacoits. Since the police were not going to do anything, Mr. Singh was planning about how to arrange the money for the ransom.

Right then, people heard sounds of shooting, which appeared to come from far. And a few seconds later, people heard the same tread of heavy feet in the backyard.

Just then, Raghu entered the room, shouting with surprise, and asking everyone to come to the backyard to see a miracle. Everyone rushed to the back of the house and saw someone lying on the stairs in the dim light of early morning. It was Sarita, motionless, perhaps asleep or not in her senses. Mr. Singh lifted her in his arms and as he was returning to the room, he saw the statue standing in its original place in the same graceful manner, to the amazement of everyone.

In a few minutes, Sarita came to her senses and she described her experience in the following words, "I do not know anything, Papa. I simply remember that those people were carrying me in the jeep and moving towards the jungle. Sometimes the moon would show up and sometimes it was all dark. I was very much afraid but I was not crying. The same fat dacoit was sitting by my side and he was driving. Another dacoit was sitting on the other side of me. Since the road was not good, the vehicle was moving slowly. We might have moved a little further, when suddenly the jeep stopped with a big jerk. The fat dacoit tried his best, but the jeep could not move at all. He shouted to the people in the other jeep and asked them to find out what the matter was. Papa, the jeep started moving backward. The fat dacoit abused the other one and asked if someone was pulling the jeep."

"Very surprising," said Mr. Singh, and he asked her to continue. "Papa, the dacoits in the other jeep clambered down and ran towards our jeep. Just then, our jeep tilted to one side and the fat dacoit fell out. Since there was no clear light, one could not see properly. I was terribly afraid now. Right then, the dacoits started shouting loudly. Some shots were fired as well. I felt as if someone had lifted me up and I was flying off. Then I do not remember. I opened my eyes only when you woke me up," Sarita said.

Suddenly, four to five people came running from the village; they appeared perplexed, and one of them started speaking, "Sir, the dacoits are lying dead in the jungle." "What!" all of them spoke at once.

The man continued, "We went for a walk in the morning towards the jungle, and we saw all the dacoits lying dead. The jeep is turned upside down."

All the people rushed to the jungle immediately. The sun was about to rise. On reaching the spot, the jeep was found to be badly crushed, like a matchbox having been crushed under the foot. One of the two dead was recognised as the chief dacoit, Madho Singh.

It was such a ghastly sight to look at the withered body of Madho Singh. His hands and legs were detached from his body, and his eyes were wide open with extreme fear, as if he had seen something extremely dangerous. His mouth was open and his teeth were protruding. Blood had flowed out from the side of the mouth. The professor felt like vomiting and Mr. Singh said, "No living person can do this." Madho Singh was holding something in his right hand. The professor removed it and found it to be a triangular piece of stone. The other jeep was lying upside down at another place. Dead bodies of all other dacoits were scattered around. They all had deep wounds on the body and fear in their eyes. Arms and ammunitions were scattered around too. Everyone was surprised to see all this and they believed that it was the act of God since no living person was capable of doing this. A man was sent to fetch the police.

On return to the building, the statue was found to have the sword, half of it matted with blood; the body had signs of bullets fired into it; the ground and the grass around appeared to have the signs of the feet of the statue; and, the top corner of the hat of the statue was found missing, which was later found to be fitting well with the triangular piece of stone, removed from the fist of the right hand of the dead dacoit Madho Singh.

The professor and Mr. Singh were surprised to imagine what could have happened. The professor advised that the statue should not be removed to the museum in the town; it could take care of itself. Mr. Singh agreed and suggested that he would spend money on the repair of the house and erect high walls around the statue for protection and converting it into a temple. Both of them agreed that it was the perfect faith of Sarita in her ancestor which caused all this to happen; and that Mr. Singh's statue saved them all. (Chakrapani 1997, March, 10-32)

Remarks

In my opinion, two things are clear from the above case: (i) Full faith, surrender and sincere prayers can invoke a soul on the higher plane, and (ii) the soul possesses all the paranormal powers which can be used in its manifestation.

Case II

Kabiruddin Sahib was born in Rangoon, Burma. He studied up to form 7 or 8 in a school there, but he was not really interested in studying. He used to go to read *namaz* (holy scripture of Muslims) but he would leave it in the middle and run away. He used to play with the vagabonds of the locality. These boys were not of good character, used to commit thefts, etc. For some time the boy Kabiruddin worked in the hotel of his father, where he was caught stealing and his father gave good beatings at times. His mother used to advise him regularly not to get involved in immoral acts and to read the holy scriptures, which would wean him away from unworthy acts. According to Kabiruddin, his mother loved him very much and used to call him Heeria with love. She wanted him to become a doctor but he had already become a thief at the early age of 12 or 13 years. It could be due to the influence of some smugglers and unwanted elements who used to come to his father's hotel. His mother was a pious lady, regular in her prayers, very graceful, but his father used to beat her also at times and Heeria did not like him.

Heeria was admitted in an English school but was removed from it after some time, since he used to run away from the school. His father used to beat him and his mother used to embrace him with love, having tears in her eyes. Burma used to have English rule at that time and Heeria used to see the devastating bombing of the Japanese everywhere. Heeria's father wanted to go to India but could not get out of Burma because of the strictness of the Japanese. However, there were many Indians doing business there. When the Japanese army entered Burma, the Indians ran away to India, leaving their flourishing businesses behind, in various groups on foot. His father was killed by dacoits on the way; they suffered several problems in the jungles of Burma for two months, but his brave mother always protected him, and they arrived in Bengal.

His mother stitched clothes for people for a livelihood and built a small house. Heeria had grown up, occupied another house left by a non-Muslim and ran a gambling house in it, unknown to his mother. When she became wise to his activities, she advised him against the opening of a gambling house, but he did not care for her and one day slapped her. She never accepted any money from his earnings. He married a prostitute, bought a car and lived a life of comforts. He started dealing in drugs. His mother prayed regularly for his change of heart.

While dealing with a Mafia group, one of his representatives was caught at the airport of a foreign country. He was carrying goods worth ten million rupees. He lost the deal with the Mafia and was lured in the trap laid by the other party, somewhere very far from his hometown. He was hung by a rope tied to his own jeep through a branch of a big tree and his body was hanging in soft mud, in which he was sinking down and down gradually. He was in the mud till his waist and his neck straightened up and it became hard like wood. He could visualise his imminent death.

Now, in the words of Kabiruddin Sahib alias Heeria himself, "Just then I saw a human shadow approaching me from the side of the small hill. The sun had set but the twilight was spread all over. Though my neck turned around, I was seeing the human shadow coming towards me. I felt that it was a woman, who had covered herself with a white sheet of cloth from top to bottom

"The woman came towards the jeep very fast. The first thing she did was to release the rope tied to the jeep. This resulted in my neck coming down. The whole weight of my body fell once again on the soft mud which began to swallow me down gradually. The woman was robed in a white sheet and her face was half covered. She threw the other end of the rope towards me and said, 'Heeria! Catch hold of the rope...'

"I was shaken to pieces. That woman was my mother. Where did my mother come from at that place? How did she come? At that time I could not think of these things. I caught hold of the rope with my hands which were still tied down. My mother began to pull the rope. God knows, where did so much strength come into her from? She pulled me out of the soft mud. As soon as I came out I fell at the feet of my mother and began to cry and sob like a child.

"My mother was moving her hand on my head with love and was saying, 'My Heeria! My Heeria! Now you must be regular in reading the *namaz.*'

"My mother supported me and carried me to the jeep. She untied the ropes from my hands and my arms. I was crying bitterly and asked her how she came to me.

"She loved me and said, 'Heeria! When you began to travel towards this area, I came to know about it. Right from that time, I began to follow you. I knew that you would not listen to me. Whatever you want to do, you will do it. Yet, mine is a mother's heart. How can I see you suffering in any way? I was afraid of the place you were going to, of those people who were against you. But on the way, you disappeared from my sight.

"I asked, 'Mother! I cannot believe it. How could you come along so far?'

"Mother replied, 'Now, do not ask this. The maidservant you had appointed for me, helped me a lot. It is good that I forgot the way to the *Dera*, and came this way towards the hill. If I would not have come here, God knows what would have happened to my son, who is like a jewel. Now, let us reach home fast.'

"I kissed the hands of my mother and said, 'Mother, I take a vow now that I will never turn to the world of crime. I will lead a pious life. I will read the *namaz* five times a day and I will serve you for the rest of my life.'

"Mother was smiling. She was loving me again and again. I seated my mother by my side in the jeep. I started the engine and began to drive in one direction hastily. I was feeling strength again in my body... On reaching the town, I did not turn towards my gambling house, rather, I drove towards our old house.

"When the house was a little distance away, my mother put her hand on mine and said, 'Heeria! Stop the car.'

"I stopped the car and asked, 'What is the matter, mother? Why have you asked me to stop the car here?' Mother opened the door of the jeep and came out of it.

"She said, 'You go home. I will meet sister Aisha and come later. I have to tell her something important.' I said, 'Well, mother, please come home soon. I am very hungry. Today, I will eat the food cooked by you.' " Mother smiled. In that smile, I sensed a desire, a disappointment. I did not think much and began to drive towards the house. On reaching home, I found that the lights were on, the door was open and people of the locality were sitting on the cots. An elderly person came and said, 'This was the wish of God.' " Even then I did not understand anything. On entering the house, I saw the housemaid began to cry and she said, 'Mother died. She took a little food in the afternoon and complained of some pain in the chest. Then, she lay down on the bed. Once she called you by name, remembered God, asked blessings for you and then she was no more.'

"My mother had died. That mother, who was with me a little while ago, who had pulled me out of that fatal soft mud and brought me up to the door of the house. I entered the room. Some women were reading something around the cot. My mother's dead body was wrapped up in a white cloth and it was lying on the cot. One of the women said, 'The nice woman remembered you a lot before dying.'

"I screamed, lost my senses and fell on the ground. I am describing the facts of life and telling you that at the time when my mother had come to the deep forest to help me out of my death, she was already dead. You may not believe me. You may be saying in your heart that I am telling a lie, but there is no need for me to assure you of the truth. I know that I am telling the truth. The time when my mother came to me, her dead body was lying on the cot in the house. What is the truth behind it? What is the secret? Neither can you find it, nor I. Let the secret remain a secret."

This was the happening narrated by Kabiruddin Sahib. His old face was bent on his chest. Tears were flowing from his eyes. He did not want to live in that town any more. His eyes were searching for his mother everywhere. He had lost his legs due to an infection. Yet, he used to crawl to the mosque five times a day to read the *namaz* according to the desire of his mother, although he was rich and had helpers to support him.

In the end, he said, "Maybe God might show mercy on me one day. He might forgive me and then mother might also forgive me." (Hamid 1997, March, 34-49)

Comments

Details have been shortened from the original text, yet enough material is retained to show the relationship of the mother to her son, especially her unconditional and deep love for him, which resulted in all the happenings. The following things are notable: (i) Mother knew telepathically the intentions of her son to go to the Mafia dealer, that the dealer had his mind changed against her son and that her son would need her help for his survival. (ii) Her desire and decision to help her son were so strong that she had to leave her body for the purpose. (iii) After leaving her body, the mother sported a body which was exactly similar to her physical body on earth in every detail, since her son believed his mother to be alive when she was helping him, until the end. (iv) The mother, in her astral form, had all the paranormal powers and she could interact with physical objects.

Case III: Journey in Time

The experiences of a person who travelled in time, two hundred years backward, from 1997 to 1797, are described in his own words, "Leaving Dileep behind, who was still engaged in prayers, I came out of the temple of Sankatamochan Mahavirji... It was afternoon. After meditation, prayers and getting the blessed food I was strolling outside. I was not sure how much time Dileep was going to take for his prayers. The time shown in my watch was 11 o'clock. I was a little hungry too. I thought of moving around a bit.

"A desire for going towards the jungle suddenly popped up in me. I had heard that several hundred years ago there was a deep forest over here. When Goswami Tulsidas established the temple, then, that is nearly three to four hundred years from now, the environment here would have been quite different. Having thoughts of this kind, I walked deep into the forest. I felt as if the forest was calling me into its depth. The more I moved inside the more I felt like going still inwards. I felt full of freshness and energy. I looked at the watch, it was 11.45. I felt like being under the spell of some magic from the forest and did not feel like going back. It was going to strike 12 noon when I thought of Dileep and turned around to go back. Just then, I heard the strong sound of thunder from somewhere. The wind began to blow strongly and the trees too began to shake. It was difficult to stand erect. I was surprised to see all this happening in the month of October. I moved quite a distance. Suddenly, I felt that I had forgotten the way. I was highly amazed to notice the deep forest which used to exist only a few hundred years ago.

"The windstorm had become quiet now. The sunny and bright atmosphere was replaced by a strange aloofness. The sound of squirrels and monkeys had disappeared. There was a pleasing smell in the atmosphere, which I could not understand. Even the sunlight filtering through the trees had some kind of redness. The time was 12.10. I noticed that I had lost much of my way within 10 to 15 minutes only. I could see a temple in front of me now. I felt as if someone called my name. It surprised me. I saw a life-size statue of goddess Kali inside the temple; a thick and long rosary of flowers was around her neck; her red tongue was out, eyes had a lustre and she was carrying a sword and a shield in her hands. Fresh flowers were scattered around. A heavy sword was hanging on the wall. I saw all this in the flash of a moment. I bowed down to the statue of the mother. Suddenly, I heard a deep voice, 'Have you come, son Ram Prasad?'

"I was astonished and I thought it was the statue speaking.

"Then, the voice came from my side, 'Look here, I am here...' I saw a sadhu sitting on a deerskin in *padmasana* (lotus posture) in the dimly lit room. "On asking the sadhu about how he knew about him, the sadhu replied, 'Ram Prasad, I have been waiting for you for such a long time. You had to come only today. Would I not know you?' On telling him that I wanted to know the direction of the Sankatamochan temple, the sadhu said, 'Going to the Sankatamochan temple was just an excuse. You had to come here only. Today is the full moon, the dark fortnight begins tomorrow.' I got worried with the situation. The sadhu appeared to be a *tantric,* six-feet-tall, strongly built, dark complexion, long and jumbled hairlocks, a red-coloured spot on the forehead, big eyes under thick eyebrows, a rosary of beads and small bones in the neck, even the ears pierced with small bones, iron bangles in the wrists and a deerskin around the waist. I was perplexed, but he had such a personality that I could not disobey him."

The sadhu told him that it was the time of Raja (king) Chet Singh and Warren Hastings and the years was 1797 and not 1997. The sadhu was performing the requirements to attain *trikal siddhi* which would give him the power to travel into the future; he already had the power to travel into the past. The author of the episode, Ram Prasad, was going to be sacrificed on the altar to please "Mother Kali" and it was for this purpose that he had been made to travel 200 years backward in time, as was told to the sadhu by Mother some time back. Ram Prasad saw Anand Narain, the minister in the kingdom, and others with him who were wearing clothes which were several hundred years old in style. He saw a very attractive young girl in the temple premises, who was called "Bhairavi". She was a virgin and was used by the sadhu for *tantric* purposes, the latter having purchased the former for a few rupees when she was a small child. Ram Prasad was tied to a tree and served a special wine, which he had to drink forcibly so that he would not create problems for the sadhu. He lost all hopes of his survival from the clutches of the sadhu. However, the girl Bhairavi, who was herself a captive with the sadhu and was looking for an opportunity to escape; killed the sadhu with the sword. She released Ram Prasad also from captivity and said, "Run away, fool."

Now, in the words of Ram Prasad, "As Bhairavi was cutting the ropes that tied me down, a sort of lightning appeared. I got the feeling that a strong thunderstorm was running outside. The lamp got extinguished, and then I lost my senses.

"When I opened my eyes, I found myself in a deep forest. I got up in alarm and astonishment, I could neither see Bhairavi, nor the *tantric* sadhu, nor the minister Anand Narain. There was no temple, but the forest all around. I came out of my astonished situation and felt as if I had been saved by some miracle. I closed my eyes and saluted Sri Sankatamochan. Undoubtedly, it has been his blessings that saved me. I started to run from there. Fortunately, I was running towards Sri Sankatamochan temple. I met Dileep on the way. He appeared perplexed. He asked me, 'Where did you go, Ram Prasad? I came out of the temple and have since been searching for you.' What could I say?

"'Brother, I was caught up in big trouble. Somehow I have been saved. But you have been searching for me since yesterday?'

"'Why since yesterday? You were in the temple a little while ago.'

"I was surprised and said, 'Since yesterday I have been under the captivity of a *tantric*. He was going to sacrifice me on the altar.'

"'What nonsense are you talking?' Dileep looked at his watch and said, 'It is hardly ten minutes ago that I came out of the temple after the prayers.'

"I also looked at my watch. Surprise! The day and date were the same, when I came to Sri Sankatamochan temple, and the time, 12.20 hours.

"What is the secret? Did I see a dream? Dileep said, 'And where did you get this rosary of red flowers from?' I was astonished and found a rosary of red flowers in my neck. It was the rosary which the *tantric* had put round my neck before putting me to sacrifice. With a jerk I threw it away. 'Oh, oh, do not throw it away,' said Dileep and he rushed to the place where the rosary had fallen, but he could not find it.

"'What is all this game?' he was very surprised. 'Just now it fell down there in front of me, and now it has disappeared!'

"I understood everything. I said, 'That rosary belonged to the time which was two hundred years ago. It has gone there. As long as it was on my body, it could be seen.'

"'I think your mind has gone out of order,' Dileep caught my hand, 'Let us go back. We have to go to the *dharmshala* (the place of stay).' 'Wait,' said I, 'Let me see, there is a temple on this side.' We entered the forest. After a long search, we found an open place. We saw a heap of broken stones and bricks. At the same place, we found a cistern made of wood. It had on it the remains of dry blood, since when, we could not say.

"'Here was that temple, my friend,' I said, 'Two hundred years! I did not see a dream. Certainly, that *tantric* was a *siddha* (adept). I had travelled into time two hundred years behind. But the poor fellow could not complete his *sadhana,* it was broken in between. His own Bhairavi...'

"Dileep caught me and started walking towards Sri Sankatamochan temple, 'Let us go and have some hot tea, only then you will come to your senses.'

"The intoxicating beauty of Bhairavi was moving in front of my eyes." (Chakrapani 1997, May, 14-22)

Comments
(i) There is a particular mental condition and environment of the surroundings under which the travel in time can take place. (ii) A long time spent in antiquity is proportional to a very small time of the present. (iii) It is extremely difficult for others to believe in the happening, except the person himself; even the relatives and close associates discard it as a fantasy. (iv) An object of the past remains visible as long as it is associated with an object of the present; as soon as that association is broken, the object of the past disappears.

General Remarks on Cases I, II and III: Hundreds of thousands of happenings of this kind have been heard and reported in India for several thousands of years. However, these three cases are from the present and their authors are still living (at the time of writing of this book).

Scientific Evidence

The phenomenon of soul is of infinite nature, and perhaps, official science will never be able to accept it, since it cannot be produced and tested in the laboratory, although it is a repeatable event. It is only the 20th century which has witnessed the invent of quantum physics, and some scientists are now beginning to believe the credibility of the soul; especially those who have had some experience of their own, and then, they try to find a connection between the two. I believe in the soul because I witnessed it a number of times myself; and, as a result of it, I resigned my position as a professor of mathematics in 1994, and my only mission left in this lifetime is to show the credible fact to the people of the world, as far as I can. *The soul is quantum, and a "quantum of something" can only be experimented upon, not the quantum itself, since it has no measure.*

Descartes, some four hundred years ago, divided the world in two clear parts – scientific and religious. And, this division will continue, since science is objective and religion is subjective. It is only a yogi, who experiences the merger of the objective and the subjective; when the seer, the seen and the seeing become one; the condition under which one experiences oneself as a soul; and this one can never deny, because it has happened to one. The level of soul can never be touched by science, even after the inter-galactic travel becomes a reality, since the "infinite" can never be encompassed by the "finite". However, quantum physics may go on giving concessions to itself, till it merges with the soul – you never know. It is fortunate that there have been and there are "path showers" in the form of saints, prophets and yogis; and, of course, science has been getting ideas from religion and the former has been following the latter, without recognising it.

As far as quantum physics goes, I would like to summarise two sets of properties which have also been quoted by Walker (1997, 133 and 134). The first one is the following set of four properties, (Goswami 1993, 9)

1. A quantum object (for example an electron) can be at more than one place at the same time (*the wave property*).
2. A quantum object cannot be said to manifest in ordinary space-time reality until we observe it as a particle (*collapse of the wave*).

3. A quantum object ceases to exist here and simultaneously appears in existence over there; we cannot say it went through the intervening space (*the quantum jump*).
4. A manifestation of one quantum object, caused by our observation, simultaneously influences its correlated twin object – no matter how far apart they are (*quantum action-at-a-distance*).

The second one is a set of *eight major existing views of quantum reality,* (Herbert 1987, 16-27)

1. There is no deep reality – from the Copenhagen School of Niels Bohr.
2. Reality is created by observation – a second part of the Copenhagen interpretation, supported by John Wheeler, Fred Wolf.
3. Reality is an undivided wholeness – the view of Walter Heitler, Fritij of Capra, David Bohem.
4. Reality consists of a steadily increasing number of parallel universes – from Hugh Everett, Paul Devies.
5. The world obeys a non-human kind of reasoning – in the mathematical logic of George Boole.
6. Neo-realism: The world is made of ordinary objects – defended by Albert Einstein, Max Planck, Louis DeBroglie, David Bohm and Erwin Shrodinger.
7. Consciousness creates reality – from Walter Heitler, Fritz London, Henry Stapp, Eugene Wigner, John von Neumann (outlandish theory with distinguished supporters).
8. The world is two-fold, consisting of potentials and actualities – says Werner Heisenberg.

According to Herbert, there are too many guesses and all of them may turn out to be wrong. Still, an answer is needed. (Herbert 1987, 27-29) And here a question is added by Claire Walker, "Will psychic sense be involved in finding it, as it is most certainly involved in comprehending the discussion?" (Walker 1987, 134) I will endeavour to answer the above questions in what follows.

I will assert once again that science follows religion, knowingly or unknowingly, and without the former recognising the latter. Almost all the points stated above have been long exploited by the religions, especially the perennial philosophy. And the scientists, having lost their grip on reality, but not publicising this state (Herbert 1987, 15), fall back to religion for clues and make their guesses. *In my opinion, a day will come when science will give up and merge into religion.* Science has already revised its fundamentals from Galileo and Copernicus to Newton; and from Newton to Einstein; and a further revision is now due in view of the quantum theory. However, a positive approach can be that science takes clues and guidance from religion and then it makes the hypothesis, theory and then the law.

The onus of proof that the soul is quantum does not lie with science, because it is not the science which has invented soul, rather, it is the religion which has been talking about the soul from time immemorial. Furthermore, it is not the science which is looking for such a proof, nor it is religion – since religion does not need a proof, it has full faith in its validity; then who is looking for such a proof? It is parapsychology which is looking for proof, because it wants to act systematically and objectively as science does. The truth is that science yet does not recognise parapsychology as science, though the parapsychologist claim it to be so and they want it to get that status. Whatever the result of this discussion may be, it is not our concern at the moment. Our concern is to show that *soul is quantum,* and the mode of proof cannot be called scientific, rather it would have to depend on "inferences and circumstantial evidences" at the best.

Volumes of information and knowledge are available through several millenniums, by way of religion and the perennial philosophy. For example, Lord Krishna, in the *Bhagavad Gita*, tells Arjun the warrior that he, and for that matter everybody else, are not the body or mind but "*Atman*" or "Soul" – which cannot be cut by a sword, cannot be dried by heat, cannot be blown by wind, cannot be wet or drowned by water, and that we all as souls have always existed, are existing and will always exist in the future. After getting this wisdom, Arjun fought and killed his erring opponents, whom he did not want to kill earlier since they were his relatives and he had an attachment to them. I need not say that these attributes of soul are of the quantum nature, since it is obvious. For more details on the attributes of *atman,* one is referred to the book on *Perennial Philosophy* by Aldous Huxley (15). When Jesus Christ says that he and his Father in heaven are one, he refers to his "High Self" which is the index of his "Soul", a permanent element and the mediator between him and God (Hall 1928, Long 1965, 32), indicating the quantum nature of soul. The concept of God to Gautama Buddha was the "Clear Light of the Void", which is described by him to have the quantum attributes.

The philosophy of the *Upanishads* was developed and enriched in the *Bhagavad Gita* and was finally systematised in *Vivek-Chudamani* (*The Crest-Jewel of Wisdom*) by Shankara in the A.D. ninth century. Some of his writings, which are illustrative of the nature of *atman*, are quoted here:

"Realise that thou art 'That' – Brahman which is untouched by the six human infirmities (hunger, thirst, greed, delusion, decay and death); *it is realised in the heart of the yogis (i.e. in samadhi), it cannot be perceived by the senses, it is imperceptible by intellect or mind.*

"*By known logical inferences and by intuition, realise thyself as Atman,* just as a meaning of a word is understood; the certainty of this truth will be established without doubt, just as water (held) in the palm of the hand."

From the quotes of Shankaracharya, who is known as the genius of Hindu philosophy, it is clear that the *atman* or soul cannot be seen through physical eyes, it can only be known through intuition or inference. That is the *basic property of a quantum object.*

Chapter 1 has the collection of information in this regard from authentic and important sources, such as, Theosophical Society, Hindu philosophy, *The Tibetan's Book of the Dead, The Egyptian's Book of the Dead*, Eckankar, the studies related to "past-life regression" by persons like Edgar Cayce and Dr. Raymond Moody, and voluminous research on out-of-body experiences by scientists like Dr. Ian Stevenson and experiences like Robert Monroe. In the first chapter, table 1 gives the seven divisions of the universe and the related description shows that after shedding the physical body, the individual travels to astral, and then to the mental plane – the lower division of which corresponds to the heaven of various religions. In that division – the individual lives in a subtle body, which can disappear at one place and simultaneously reappear at another place, which can converse telepathically with another entity, whatever the distance between them and with no force or energy required, which can change clothes as one likes or even change shape as one likes, and which has some other attributes too, all of which taken together, exceed the four quantum properties enumerated by physicist Amit Goswami. Thus, quantum physicists have several clues to test and establish the further properties of the quantum. In the hierarchy of planes of the universe, when the individual upgrades to the next intuitive plane after the mental plane, even the subtle body is left behind and one lives now as the "formless soul", and then, still higher properties of the quantum nature are encountered.

Next, we come to the field of psychology and parapsychology on one hand and yoga and meditation on the other. The present chapter has been specially devoted to the study of the ego and self through dreams by Carl Jung, and the study of *atman* or self and *Sat-Chit-Ananda* through yoga and meditation by Sri Aurobindo. Carl Jung has shown that ego is the centre of the phenomenal world while self is the centre of the whole psyche. Ego takes care of the outer personality while self takes care of the inner personality. According to him, self is a sub-set of psyche – which is "whole". *Psyche* is universal, collective, eternal, unique, a cosmic principle and existence itself. According to Sri Aurobindo, ego is the centre of "surface mind", while the *psychic being* is the centre of the "subliminal". He divided self into two parts – *Jivatma* and Psychic Being. While *jivatma,* as a portion of the Divine, is universal as well as individual, the psychic being narrows to sheer individuality. Thus, *jivatma* or *atman* is the permanent element for which Jung said that it is of the size less than a thumb and at the same time covers the whole universe. Sufi saint Meher Baba also said that when the unconscious is brought to the conscious, it is the realisation of the eternal element which can be called "soul"; the orthodox religions call it God. (Baba 1967) So, the "Psyche" of Jung, "Atman" of Sri Aurobindo, or "Soul" of Meher Baba are quantum in nature, having properties much more than what the quantum physics has discovered till now.

Next, three true-life cases presented earlier which are the index of hundreds of thousands of cases happened in the past few millenniums, evince the quantum property of the soul. Innumerable yogis from all over the world have reported being on higher realms in their soul body exhibiting quantum properties; see for example, *Twentieth-Century Mystics and Sages* by Anne Bancroft (1976). Lastly, I would reproduce a brief account of one of my own experiences (Kumar 1994), which I had in the year 1987, soon after witnessing the awakening of *kundalini.*

"I found myself standing in front of a translucent fortress which had a canal of clear blue water running at the middle of it. On both sides of the canal there were gates; people were entering from the left gate and coming out of the right one. People were moving slowly in a queue. Persons there were in the form of invisible points, having semi-circular auras of light around them; it was because of the aura that they could be seen or recognised. I was standing up in the sky and I could see three persons near the ground talking to each other. After a while, I got some instructions in my being from one of the persons near the ground, telling me to move forward. The moment I decided to leave the place, I found myself in another location which had green meadows, trees and lakes around, and a pleasing bluish-green light was lighting the area, but the light had no source.

"I was fully conscious of my being there. Suddenly, I looked around myself and I wanted to see my constitution. I noticed that I had no hands, legs or any part of a physical body – I was just there. I could see in all directions simultaneously. I was filled with the feeling of happiness and bliss and was slowly moving towards a big river or a canal of clear blue water; it was so wide that it looked like an ocean. I was going in a straight line and it appeared to be a bridge having the width of a hair, but nothing visible. It was a wonderful experience till I crossed the water and was on the opposite bank. There, I saw a group of mountains and as soon as I approached close to one of them, I returned to my physical body on earth.

"I had several dreams, visions and out-of-body experiences for a few months, especially in that year 1987."

I can confirm with my experiences that the soul is an invisible point of existence, it can disappear at one place and appear simultaneously at another just by way of thinking, it can communicate with another soul telepathically – questions and answers emerging in the being and we recognise each other through intuition. These are quantum properties of the soul. Perhaps, other properties of quantum nature can be gathered through a review of other experiences – my own and those of several others.

Conclusion

There has been overwhelming evidence to the fact that *atman or soul is not only the non-local aspect of human beings but it is fully quantum in nature.* Rather, the quantum has yet to evolve in its fullness to acquire the properties of the soul. Religion, psychology / parapsychology and individual cases – all of them have testified to the above. However, the proof is based on circumstantial evidence and intuition, not on laboratory tests, because the soul can only be observed through intuition. In fact, the onus would have been on the "quantum" of physics to prove that it has the properties of the "soul", and not the other way round. But alas, the scientists – even though they follow guidance from religion, knowingly or unknowingly – never pay proper respect to it. And this is the reason that, in spite of tremendous achievements made by science, there is no peace in the hearts of the people. Not only the galactic colonisation appears to become a reality in the near future, but other feats, such as reducing man to the size of a cockroach and vice versa, disappearance of man at one place and reappearance at another, etc. may come up on the scene of the world; yet, competition, fear, jealousy and unhappiness will prevail in the society. This is because of the non-recognition of the religion. That slowly people are turning towards "meditation" and "looking inwards" is not by choice but by compulsion. In my opinion, the best way would be a synthesis of science and religion, since both are necessary for evolution and an all-round development of human, but when it would happen is anybody's guess.

I will now turn to the questions posed by physicist Herbert and Claire Walker with respect to the eight major existing views of quantum reality. The second part of the Copenhagen interpretation of Niels Bohr that reality is created by observation appears to be correct, in association with point number seven, that consciousness creates reality. As described in Chapter 1, and supported by the findings of Jung and Sri Aurobindo in Chapter 2, the universe has various divisions, according to the level of consciousness. The most acceptable number of divisions at present is seven. Just as a bottle of water having in it stone pieces, sand, ash and water will appear to have only stones if the viewer has a solid, physical viewpoint of observation, or it will have only water if the observer has only the liquid for test in his mind, even so, everything in the world exists and the reality will depend on the consciousness of the observer. A man sitting in a restaurant and simultaneously eating food and reading a book, may not really know the taste of the food if he is deeply observed in reading the book. Even the horn of a car in the street, the smell of roses in the garden around and the biting of a mosquito in the arm may be non-realities for him since he is not conscious of them, although they do really exist. Suddenly, a loud horn may distract his attention from reading and eating, and at that time, noise is the only reality he may be living in. Similarly, a purely worldly person lives and knows the reality of the physical world only; a man of meditation may be living in the realities of the astral world, although the physical world exits around him; and a saint or a prophet may be living the reality of cosmic bliss of soul, although both physical and astral worlds are around him. Even in the affairs of the world, someone with a happy disposition will find that everyone in the world is happy, since his attention is attracted by happy people only. A person with gloomy attitude may conclude that everyone in the world is unhappy, since his attention is attracted by unhappy people only. The world appears to be of the same colour as the colour of the glasses of the observer.

The first part of Copenhagen interpretation, that there is no deep reality, is not fully agreeable with me since the knowledge is endless and there is always one more step to know, whatever the level of knowledge may be. God has infinite attributes, and in Hinduism we say that even if the whole surface of the world is used as paper and the whole ocean is used as ink, the attributes of God cannot be covered. Niels Bohr may be right if he is concerned with the realities known to man so far, but he is wrong if he talks about the realities in general, since there is much more unknown than is known. Point number three, that the reality is an undivided wholeness, seems to be correct since this is what all religions have been saying and it is also the experience of the saints and self-realised thinkers.

Point number four needs a careful assessment. That reality has an increasing number of parallel universes is true in the sense that everyday a new universe is being discovered. But the number of universes in reality as a whole may be fixed, it is only us who come to know the truth gradually. A new star being discovered adds to the library of physics, but there may be infinitely many which are not yet known to physics. Thus, the library of physics is steadily increasing. However, in religion, we are told that new universes are created and destroyed continuously by the Ultimate Reality, so there may not be a fixed number in this regard.

Point number five is seemingly correct since the human reasoning is of the finite nature (as the whole reality is not known to him) and the universe is obeyed by laws beyond human thinking. Paranormal happenings, such as telepathy, telekinesis, precognition and levitation are beyond human reasoning.

Point number six, that the world is made of ordinary objects, may be true as far as the physical world is concerned.

Point seven, that consciousness creates reality is perfectly correct and covered earlier.

Point eight, that the world is twofold, consisting of potentials and actualities is also correct. In fact, the Ultimate Reality has two divisions, as pointed out by religion – potential and kinetic. Potential energy corresponds to the static state of *Satchidananda*, the sleeping storehouse, and the kinetic energy is responsible for the creation of the universe and its objects, *kundalini* being a name given to it in Hinduism.

However, the psychic sense will certainly be involved in finding the answers related to the quantum reality, if one wants to have a direct intuitive knowledge of the facts, and then one would be able to talk with an authority. Otherwise, one can draw inferences after a lot of research and yet not be confident of what one is talking about. This is why Herbert said that all the eight views on quantum reality could be wrong. This uncertainty is due to the fact that the scientists have not seen the reality intuitively, which they are postulating theoretically. Hence, the necessity of the psychic sense.

Summary: The views proposed towards the quantum reality are not in conflict with each other, rather they appear to exist simultaneously. They could be guesses based on certain observations. The details of life on the seven divisions of the universe, as presented in Chapter 1, can give constructive ideas for research to the physicists and other scientists in general. It is quite possible that these views have been formed only after seeing the literature which has been the basis for Chapter 1, for example, the Theosophical Society, *The Tibetans Book of the Dead* or the cases of past-life regression. However, there are a large number of properties that can be found to be associated with a quantum object. I would suggest the following.

Parallel to the soul, a quantum object may have the following properties:

i) *Self-existent:* A quantum object, for example, an electron, is the most basic unit of existence which is not a product or resultant of any process, and every other thing is made of it, there is nothing that is made but not made of it in the universe.

Hence a quantum object is self-existent.

This property is suggested by the "perennial philosophy" which says that God is the only doer; Its kinetic part of energy, which is of the quantum nature, is the creator of everything that exists in the universe; see, for example, the *Bhagavad Gita.* And in the *Bible* too, we read, "In the beginning was the Word, and the Word was with God, and the Word was God, everything that was created was created by the Word, there is nothing which was not created by Word." Thus, Word is the "quantum energy unit" of God.

ii) *Most Basic Unit:* A quantum object, being the most basic unit of existence, cannot be cut or divided further, cannot be dried, cannot be wet and it cannot be blown by any kind of known forces. It is a permanent element of existence.

iii) *Omnipresent*: The first and the third properties stated by physicist Amit Goswami, combined in one, would mean a quantum object can be at more than one place at the same time and it may cease to exist at one place and reappear at another, without going through the intervening space. This means that a quantum object, of its own will, may appear anywhere at any time and at more than one place simultaneously, that is, it can be found anywhere or everywhere. This is the property of omnipresence attributed to God alone; but since soul is akin to God, the soul also has this property.

The astral plane, the second from the lowest in the hierarchy of seven divisions of the universe, has the property that an individual can appear anywhere at any time in its astral body. This is how you see the dead relatives around you a few days before your death. On the astral plane, the moment you think of being with a person, either you are with him or he is with you in no time. This is because astral bodies are made of quantum elements.

On the mental plane, next to the astral, whose lower division is called heaven in orthodox religions, the property of omnipresence is much more well defined, since the mental body is made of yet finer vibrations than those of the astral plane.

Hence a quantum object is omnipresent.

iv) *Omnipotence*: Astral people can create food of their liking just by thinking about it; and for that matter, clothes, vehicles, houses, flowers and any other thing which they want to have, can be produced instantaneously. They can call any person to them, they can go anywhere (of course on the astral and physical planes), and they can, in fact, create a world of their own – are these not the properties of omnipotence? And, the people at the mental plane have this faculty much more well defined. It is further well defined on the intuitive plane, which is higher than the mental, and so on.

The tremendous energy produced by the disintegration of an atom is given by the formula: $E = 1/2\ m\ c^2$, which is just an example of the action at the quantum level. Another example is the power of the laser beams which can cut through steel. More similar uses of the energy at the quantum level will be developed by science in the future. Finally, physics is going to conclude that:

A quantum object is omnipotent.

v) *Omniscient*: People on the astral and higher planes, in increasing order, of course, have the capability of knowing about what is happening anywhere on their plane or on a plane lower than theirs, instantly. Thus, a person on the mental plane, which is known as the abode of saints and seers, can know instantly about anything happening anywhere on the mental, astral or physical plane. The quantum nature of the persons belonging to the mental plane is much more uncovered with regard to ego-pollution. Thus, God, who is higher than the highest imaginable plane, is, no doubt, fully omniscient. The degree of omniscience increases from the lowest plane onwards in a gradual manner. This would suggest that:

A quantum object is omniscient.

The Phenomenon of Identification

Each one of us has infinite potentialities as a soul. But we are confined into the narrowness and limitations of this physical body, which most of us consider to be the only reality. Thus, it is the identification of the soul with the body which limits us. When we are driving a car, we can move faster – this is identification with the car. And when we are flying in an aeroplane, we can move still faster, since then we have identified ourselves with the aeroplane. If, however, we can identify ourselves with the self within or the soul, we can move with the speed of the thought, because then we, as souls, have the quantum properties. Nevertheless, identification with a car or an aeroplane is easy, but identification with the soul is not so easy, although not impossible either. This identification with soul is called "individuation" by Jung, "transformation" by Sri Aurobindo, and Self-realisation by most of the saints and some orthodox religions. Irrespective of whatever faith or religion one has, the process of identification with the soul awakens a sleeping power within the individual, or, perhaps, it would be right to say that the awakening of the sleeping power brings the identification with the soul. The most popular name for this sleeping power is *kundalini*. The next chapter is concerned with various methods of transformation and an introduction to this power.

3
TRANSFORMATION AND KUNDALINI

Planes of Inner Reality

Sri Aurobindo has divided the Inner Reality into the following planes of existence, from the highest to the lowest:

1. *Plane of Existence, Consciousness and Bliss* (*Sat-Chit-Ananda*) – *Brahman.*
2. *Plane of Supermind,* real centre of the totality of our being.
3. *Plane of Overmind,* the direct descent of the supermind, intermediary between knowledge and ignorance, "a suprconscient cosmic Mind in direct contact with the Supramental Truth-Consciousness, an original intensity determinant of all movements below it and all mental energies". (Sri Aurobindo 1970, 333)
4. *Plane of Intuition,* a special formation of the overmind – sudden and intimate flash of self-existent knowledge – Truth-vision, Truth-thought, Truth-sense, Truth-feeling, Truth-action.

5. *Plane of Illumined Mind*, one of vision, truth-sight and truth-light, "it illumines the thought-mind with a direct vision and inspiration, brings a spiritual light and energy into its feelings and emotion". (Sri Aurobindo 1970, 1124-1125)
6. *Plane of Higher Mind*, just above the conscious mind, "spiritual parent of our conceptive mental ideation... a unitarian sense of being with a powerful multiple dynamisation capable of the formation of a multitude of aspects of knowledge, ways of action, forms and significance of becoming, of all of which there is a spontaneous inherent knowledge". (Sri Aurobindo 1970, 1118)
7. *Plane of Conscious Mind*, when "pure consciousness" descends from above, it gets mixed up with "ignorance" gradually, and its purity, comprehension and force are diminished. Conversely, when the evolution takes place, the individual consciousness passes from the lowest level of "conscious mind" to the higher mind, and gets on gathering more and more purity, comprehension and force in the ascending order of the planes.

One can compare the above seven planes with the seven planes of Chapter 1 – the division of the universe (Table 1):

	Chapter 1		*Sri Aurobindo*
1.	Divine	________	*Satchidananda*
2.	Monadic	________	Supermind
3.	*Atmic*	________	Overmind
4.	Intuitional	________	Intuition
5.	Mental	________	Illumined Mind
6.	Astral	________	Higher Mind
7.	Physical	________	Conscious Mind

One can see the parallelism between the two modes of division. A natural hypothesis would be, that, as the consciousness of the individual becomes higher, he belongs to the next plane. Thus, an individual with a conscious mind only is a person of the physical type living also on the physical plane. A person with a higher mind belongs to the astral plane, although living on the physical plane. This class might include people who can exhibit paranormal powers while living on earth. A person possessing an illumined mind belongs to the mental plane, yet living on earth. One can proceed like this unto the utmost division.

According to Sri Aurobindo, the various grades of division, which actually correspond to the energy-substance of the spirit, do really exist and there are worlds corresponding to all of them. *Satchidananda* (*Sat-Chit-Ananda*) is Itself the potential Energy while Its kinetic energy-substance, which he calls Consciousness-Force, assumes different forms of energy on different planes of existence. Thus, it is psychic energy of the psychic being, mental energy of the mind, vital energy of the vital body, and physical energy of the physical body. With its descent into the lower planes, the subtlety of this force converts into grossness, and loses its purity, comprehension and universality. It is the will of the Transcendent Spirit, called "tapas" by him, which brings the manifestation of the individual on various planes. However, in the inner subtle form, the force is universal, while in the outer gross form, it is individual – with all its limitations. The inner being is relatively unchangeable and "knows itself in time, in the present, past and future, but at once, with an undivided view which embraces all the mobile experiences of the Time-self". (Sri Aurobindo 1970, 603-604) In his opinion, desire is the deformation of will in the dominant bodily life and physical mind. "The essential turn of the soul to possession and enjoyment consists in a will to delight." (Sri Aurobindo 1970, 695-696) Thus, *delight* is the "pure form of requirement" by the soul, while *desire* is the deformation of this requirement which manifests in the form of worldly pleasures.

Spiritual Dynamics and Kundalini

The *inner reality* has two poles – the lower part is exterior, instinctive, surface or conscious mind, while the higher part is interior, archetypal self or spiritual psychic being – according to Jung and Sri Aurobindo, respectively. The exterior centre is personal, individualistic, and a product of the outside world, while the interior centre is transpersonal, universal and fundamental. The exterior centre is formed by the dynamics of the interior centre on the pattern of the latter. "But there is another side of the structure regarding which Jung makes only wild guesses, while Sri Aurobindo presents a well-knit view. It is the vertical elevation of the inner reality." (Singh 1986, 139) The inner reality elevated vertically has a height; Sri Aurobindo calls it "self", which is a fundamental entity in itself and the psychic being is a representative of it. Jung, on the other hand, considers self to be only a part of the psyche.

The words "energy" and "force" have been used by both the thinkers for both the physical and spiritual parts of the reality. However, Jung calls the 'intuitive' side 'energy' and the 'physical' side 'force'; while Sri Aurobindo calls the 'spiritual principle of creation' 'Consciousness-Force' and 'evolutionary process' 'energy'. Jung has tried to extend the scientific concept of energy to the field of inner reality, with the difference that quantity is replaced by quality, as pointed out earlier. Sri Aurobindo, on the other hand, makes use of the term 'force'. According to him, (i) consciousness is inherent in the "Consciousness-Force", wherever it manifests itself, (ii) before manifestation the force undergoes the process of involution, and (iii) it is the pull of the 'self' exerted on its own involved forms or the psychic being which results in the manifestation of various psychic forces during evolution. Jung, too, has invariably maintained that consciousness is a part of the unconscious, and hence consciousness and energy are the two fundamentals of the inner reality. Then, according to him, it is the 'residue of experiences' by the organism which forms the collective unconscious and the 'psyche'. These *experiences,* which would have been *conscious* at the time of their taking place with the organism, are now lying *dormant* in the unconscious and constantly trying to *re-emerge* on the surface. According to Jung, this attempt of re-emergence of the dormant experiences is the main source of psychic energy; while according to Sri Aurobindo, the involution began from the monotheistic *Satchidananda.* Lastly, Jung considers the psychic force emerging from the tension between the instinctive and the archetypal parts of the psyche, as compared to Sri Aurobindo's observation that it is the pull of the self on the "psychic being" which resulted in the formation of the psychic force.

The Kundalini

According to Sri Aurobindo, the spiritual dynamics is the Consciousness-Force which is inherent in *Satchidananda* as the source of all creation. The same Force is inherent in the self and its representative 'psychic being', which emanated from *Satchidananda.* The *Consciousness-Force,* which may now be called the *psychic force,* goes into the hiding behind the veil of the mental, vital and physical, and it lies *dormant* there after all the creation. The situation has its parallelism in Jung's findings when he says that the *residue of experiences* are lying *dormant* in the unconscious. The dormant "Consciousness-Force" of Sri Aurobindo or the "residue of experiences" of Jung is the *Kundalini* of *Tantra* which lies dormant in the root centre called *muladhara chakra* after the creation. The "upward surge" of the "psychic force" with the evolution of the world is the "rising and ascension" of the *kundalini* in *tantra*. As the psychic force, on evolution, passes through the physical, vital, mental and supramental planes, the *kundalini* passes through the various centres of energy called the *chakras*. It is important to note that corresponding to the seven planes of the universe of Sri Aurobindo, there are seven *chakras* through which the *kundalini* has to pass. They are: *muladhara, swadhishthan, manipura, anahata, vishuddhi, ajna* and *sahasrara,* in the ascending order. One can see the truth of the statement, "as above so below" – there are seven planes in the universe, and there are seven *chakras* in the human body, from the base of the root of the spine to the crown of the head. As the *kundalini* rises from the first to the seventh centre, the individual consciousness rises from the lowest physical plane to the highest plane of *Satchidananda*. Man is the replica of the universe, and so, the macro-process of the universe is also going on as micro-process in the human body, in exactly the same way. For *tantric* details of the *kundalini* and the seven *chakras,* the reader is referred to my book, *Journey Back To Our True Home – Through Spiritual Energy Kundalini.* (Kumar 1998)

Orthodox religion says that soul is a universal entity and it is not concerned with the individualistic side of the person. But both Sri Aurobindo and Jung believe that soul is both individualistic and universalistic. According to them, the external individualistic behaviour is certainly connected with the core of the subconscient or unconscious. The universality, according to Jung, is due to the collective unconscious which has been developed since the beginning of the organic life and it is a "common property" inherited by all humans. According to Sri Aurobindo, universality is the essential attribute of all souls since they have emanated from the same *Satchidananda*. It is camouflaged by the ego. The moment the ego is eradicated, the psychic being, which is the representative of the soul, displays universality. So this is one point where the two geniuses are one and they differ from the orthodox belief.

Sri Aurobindo believed that we live simultaneously on various planes, which are physical, vital, mental and supramental. And, correspondingly, our supramental, mental and vital growth is transmitted through the physical body, along with certain hereditary traits from birth to birth. This is because of the embodiment of the psychic traits in the mental, mental in the vital and the vital in the physical. It is important to note here that a similar conclusion was drawn in Chapter 1, which confirms this fact. We had observed there that the causal body on its downward journey gathers the mental, astral and physical bodies in that order, and this complete embodiment is called the "personality" of the individual. Thus, according to Sri Aurobindo, the total preformed personality, along with certain hereditary traits, is transmitted to the individual at the time of rebirth. He was very clear and undoubtful about this transmission. Jung, on the other hand, believed on "heredity being the sole carrier" and was puzzled and bewildered by the idea that spirituality and universality could be transmitted through human genes, which are only of the physical nature. Heredity, in view of Sri Aurobindo, was only a subordinate factor. To continue, both researchers believed in the simultaneous existence of the physical and the psychic, without either of them depending on the other, as a set of coordinate entities. However, about the ultimate nature of the "inner reality", Jung was dubious and speculative only, while Sri Aurobindo was certain. Sri Aurobindo believed that "matter" and "psychic being" were the manifestations of the "existence" and "delight" attributes, respectively, of *Satchidananda* Itself.

Method of Individuation

The "whole" has been divided into pieces and this is the cause of the miseries of the human beings. Integration of the divisiveness is therefore required. Instinctive divisiveness could be overcome by the integration of ego which resulted in the stability of humans in the world. Now the ego has taken over the conscious mind and it is over-playing its role. The egoistic divisiveness should now be integrated so that the conscious and the unconscious are combined into one whole psyche. Self is that higher principle, found by Jung, which can bring about this integration by the process called "individuation".

Patients of Jung, suffering from diseases like neurosis or schizophrenia, dreamt of circular images such as coiled snakes or circular race of fish when they were cured and satisfied. Such images are called *mandala* and Jung regards them stronger archtyepal than anima or animus of any kind. Since the *mandala* appeared in the state of unconsciousness and it reconciled the problems of ego, Jung said that "it signifies the wholeness of the self". Individuation is "the process by which a person becomes a psychological 'in-dividual'. That is, a separate indivisible unity or 'whole'" (Jung n.d. 1, IX, I, 275) According to Dr. Chaturbhuj Sahai, "When the *ray* of Brahmic power descends down from its abode for creation, it stops at five places in the universe and makes the *mandala*. ...In these *mandalas,* five elements – earth, water, fire, air and *akash* – are present in variations, but one of the elements remains prominent as compared to remaining others. Because of the presence of these five elements, every *mandala* has a distinct form, colour, work, sound and light. Although the light and sound is one, but because of the interactions of the elements, it appears to be having different forms. Removal of these variations and bringing oneself to the unity in one, is called 'practise and *sadhana*'. The same *ray* is called *kundalini* by yogis, *surti* by saints and '*rooh-va-tavajjah*' by the Muslim Sufis'. (Sahai 1987, 603)

Conscious mind functions in the waking state, while the unconscious functions in the sleeping state. Accordingly, we all are dual personalities. And again, the unconscious has a personal and an impersonal unconscious, formed by the experiences of the individual and the race respectively. Ego can take care of either the conscious or the unconscious, because of its divergent nature. Hence, some unconscious formation at a time cannot be taken care of by the ego, and this is the cause of the division of personality. The alternation of the other personality with the usual one leads the individual to a pathological state. A large number of such cases are found in the West today. Cure of such a state requires the unification of the conscious and the unconscious. Analysing the dreams of his patients, Jung found that a point could be located in the psyche of the individual which would unite the divergent elements. But "as opposites never unite at their own level, a supraordinate 'third' is always required, in which the two parts can come together". (Jung n.d. 1, IX, II, 180)

Since a total alteration of ego may result in a chaotic condition, Jung recommends the maintenance of a strong ego which can withstand the impact of the unconscious; and, by a close contact of the 'strong ego' with the 'self', let the former realise its subordinate position compared with the latter. The contact can be developed by assimilating more and more contents of the unconscious by the ego. This would serve two purposes – bringing the unconscious into the conscious, and the ego is shifted from its place and there is a change in its attitude. Gradually, the personality is enlarged by the unconscious and the ego is dwarfed. An uncompromising and stubborn attitude of the ego has shifted and it accepts the subordination to the "stronger factor, namely to the new totality-figure, that is, 'self'". (Jung n.d. 1, viii, 25) However, a danger is that if the ego is very strong, it may impersonate as self after the shifting of the centre. History is replete with such people who exercise ego in the name of the self and engage themselves in selfish acts. Another problem which can arise is in case the ego is weak and unable to withstand the impact of the unconscious. In such a case, the ego goes back to "preconscious wholeness" and the confusion derails the person from individuation. The ego gets weakened and it "gives rise to a sort of nebulous superman with a puffed-up ego and a deflated self". (Jung n.d. 2, 225) Accordingly, Jung advises the maintenance of ego while searching for the self, and let the former realise its relatively lower position in comparison with the latter in a natural way.

Anima and animus are the contents of the unconscious corresponding to the feminine and masculine parts, respectively, into which the ego is divided. These feminine and masculine aspects of the ego are represented by sentimental and intellectual aspects of the consciousness, respectively. Thus, man's consciousness is dominated by intellectuality and the unconscious by anima; and, the woman's consciousness is dominated by sentiments and the unconscious by animus. Whenever a balance is reached between the female and male aspects of the nature, the woman or man becomes androgynous and individuation is achieved. I have already gone into deeper details on this aspect of the nature. (Kumar 1997)

Involvement in the emotional ties loosens the grip on the objectivity in life. Thus, emotional ties prove to be a big obstacle on the way to individuation. According to Jung, "If we can visualise an undercurrent of objectivity even behind the emotional ties, and disengage it from within the subjectivity even behind the emotional ties, and disengage it from within the subjective projections, we would be on a sure way to individuation. The person, who has attained psychic wholeness is, immune to emotional disturbance and subjective bias." (Singh 1986, 156)

On achieving "wholeness" as a fruit of individuation the person may come across numinous objects in dreams and visions, such as, religious or lofty human personalities and signs of cross, circle, duality, etc. which may indicate the completion of the process. Jung does not like to give a spiritual status to the person at this stage; however, he considers such a perfected person to be ideal for the society for the development of the civilisation as a whole. "Through the process of individuation, an individual first returns to the 'fundamental facts of his own being' and thus becomes 'conscious of his distinctiveness'." (Singh 1986, 157)

Jung considers humans to be of two types – extrovert and introvert; and, the human nature has four functions – sensation, feeling, thinking and intuition. Thus, there are *eight kinds of people* altogether, ranging from sensing extrovert to intutiting introvert. An extrovert is predominated by objective considerations, and he considers subjectivity to be a disturbing element. An introvert thinks that an object is only a representative of the subjective content; and, self and subjective psychological process are above any object. Normally, both mechanisms work in an individual corresponding to outer circumstances and inner dispositions. A disbalance brings a pathological state, and a perfect balance is a rare thing. Jung prefers introversion to extroversion, since too much interest in the objective world finally leads to ego-centralism and the person may lie anywhere from childish selfishness to wickedness and brutality. An introvert may also develop a wrong attitude but it is not so common. In a neurotic person, for example, ego may start functioning as self due to excessive subjectivity unknowingly, which can bring chaotic results.

Method of Transformation

Sri Aurobindo divides evolution into three stages: ascension, integration and *tapas*. Ascension is a radical development from one grade of consciousness to another, for example from physical to vital, from vital to mental, and so on. Integration is a consolidation of the quantitative change in one particular grade. *Tapas* is the concentration of a particular stage into the formation of the self. Even after millions of years of evolution, man is not yet free from physical, vital and instinctive constraints. "Physical incapabilities, habitual constraints, instinctive compulsions, emotional pressures and ideological conflicts pull him down or keep him in conflict... Advent of seer after seer, sage after sage, prophet after prophet is, at least, demonstrative of the will of man to formulate and reformulate certain basic ideas so as to make them more and more effective in improving the behaviour of man... Ideals of Buddha, Christ and others have been institutuionalised. After initial impact, of course, all institutions have degenerated into dead structures." (Singh

1986, 161-162) The reason, according to Sri Aurobindo, is that the inner reality is made of many inner states corresponding to various planes, which actually exist and are connected organically with one another. One, therefore, needs an integral transformation of the complete set of states, not only the conscious mind which is only the outer state.

According to Sri Aurobindo, "At present, the soul or Self in us, intent on indiviualisation in Nature, allows itself to be confused with the idea of the ego... (hence) a deliverance form the limiting an imprisoning ego is the first elementary step towards the being of the gnosis. (However, the ego is) our rock of safety against the cosmic and the infinite. It is, therefore, small wonder that no sooner one gets rid of the ego, one finds oneself 'dissolved in a vast impersonality'. This is, by no means, a welcome state of things. It does not only stand on the brink of eclipsing the individuality of the person but also makes him bereft of the 'key to an ordered dynamism of action' " (Singh 1986, 163) Thus, on one hand, the ego is to be eradicated, and on the other, it is required to save our individuality. So what is the way out of this paradoxical situation? The only way out is to shift the centre of personality from the ego to the self. But the self is not directly available; it can be approached only through its representative "psychic being", which is itself trying to reach its originator transcendent self. Hence, the shift has to be in two stages – firstly, from ego to psychic being, and secondly, from psychic being to the self. The following steps are suggested for the same:

1. Relieve the physical of its sense of 'limitation'. This is achieved by the realisation that physical is nothing but the concretised form of the vital. This leads to the expansion of the physical into the vital.

2. Relieve the vital of its characteristic feature, 'desire'. Desires have caused the formation of instincts. Furthermore, unfulfilled and suppressed desires have gone into the subconscious and formed a screen which is strong enough to appear as the centre of personality, erroneously. This screen is nothing but another form of ego.
3. Pierce the mental sheath, which is the result of selective outer experiences, and go behind it. Direct entry of the conscious mind into the subconscious is not recommended since "it would plunge us into incoherence or into sleep or a dull trance or a comatose torpor". (Sri Aurobindo 1970, 266) One should enter first into the subliminal or ascend the superconscient. This requires one to purify the surface nature and then explore all regions of the subconscient – physical, vital and mental – through the enhanced power of one's knowledge. Suppression of subconscious can misfire the whole thing. One requires the *illumination* of the "whole subconscious" by *some higher consciousness.* Any part of it which is not transformed can nullify the whole thing. "Only when no part of the consciousness makes any response to these forces of the lower plane, then the victory and transformation are absolutely complete." (Sri Aurobindo 1958, III, 899) This would establish the individual fully in the psychic being and the subliminal as a whole.

Thus, psychic transformation is affected in two phases: (i) purification of the physical, sublimation of the vital and enlargement of the surface mind; and (ii) enlightenment of the subconscious by a higher consciousness of the psyche. The physical and the vital are transformed and the mind is universalised by illumination; weaknesses are eradicated and the life is charged with the Consciousness-Force; and, the outer personality also extends itself beyond its body and inhabits the body of the universe.

According to Sri Aurobindo, an important principle of the world is "duality". He has defined the two poles as follows:

i) Pole one: Outer Physical;
Pole two : Inner Physical – which provides the substance not only of our physical, but vital and mental sheaths too.

ii) Pole one: Outer Vital – involved in the physical body, bound by its past evolution in Matter;
Pole two : Inner Vital – a subliminal force of life which is not boxed between the narrow boundaries of vital being behind the form of living, which we ignorantly take for our real existence.

iii) Pole one: Surface Mind – of our expressed evolutionary ego, the superficial mentality created by us in our emergence out of Matter;
Pole two: Subliminal Mind – which is not hampered by our actual mental life and its strict limitations, something large, powerful and luminous, the true mental being behind that superficial form of mental personality which we mistake for ourselves.

iv) Pole one: Surface Desire-Soul – which works in our vital cravings, our emotional aesthetic faculty and mental seeking for power, knowledge and happiness;
Pole two : Subliminal Psychic Entity – a pure power of light, love, joy and refined essence of being which is our true soul behind the outer form of psychic existence.

v) Pole one: Complex of Outer Physical, Vital, Mental and Psychic – an individuality which is operative in our ordinary life and, which is egoistic in its central principle;
Pole two: Complex of Inner Physical, Vital, Mental and Psychic – which is characterised as our 'Larger

> True Individuality', and is psychic. It is close to our universality, touches it, is in constant relation and commerce with it – "psychic personality", the development of which is the goal of all our evolution in consciousness. (Sri Aurobindo 1970, 262-264; 1958, I, 288, Singh 1986, 168-169)

Sri Aurobindo defined two systems of existence: concentric and vertical. The "psychic being" is the centre of the concentric inner reality only, while the totality of our being, which is composed of several vertically superimposed planes, is circumspected by the "superconscient". His comparison can be tabled as follows:

egoistic consciousness	______________	a flickering lamp
psychic consciousness	______________	moon
superconscient	______________	sun

It is the superconscient which illumines the whole system, and "the mind's formulae dissolve in a white flame of direct inner experience" when one reaches the supramental consciousness. The superconscient "may form itself as a spiritualised intuitive light and power in the mind itself". These are the signs of gnostic or spiritual transformation, achieved by concentration on heart-centre with love, *bhakti* (devotion) and surrender; which, removes the soul or psychic being from its hiding to govern body, life and mind, and "open them fully to the Divine". While "the power of concentration above the head is to bring peace, silence, liberation from the body sense, the identification with mind and life opens the way for the lower (mental, vital, physical) consciousness to rise up to meet the higher consciousness above and for the powers of the higher (spiritual nature) consciousness to descend into mind, life and body". (Sri Aurobindo 1958, II, 725) "For making these transformations possible, what we have to do is to take hold of the 'exterior being' and make it an instrument of the Divine. This can be done by remembering the Divine constantly and at the same time by opening our nature upward so as to facilitate the descent. This is to be supplemented by 'constant faith and reliance on the Mother'." (Singh 1986, 170)

This type of a person is determined by the principle which lies at the centre of one's personality. The three types whose consciousness is related to the surface mind, are described by Sri Aurobindo, in the ascending order of consciousness, as follows:

1. *Physical Man,* mainly occupied with his corporeal life and habitual needs, impulses, life habits, mind habits, body habits, looking very little or not at all beyond that, subordinating and restricting all his other tendencies and possibilities to that narrow formation.

2. *Vital Man,* concerned with self-affirmation, self-aggrandisement, self-enlargement, satisfaction of ambition, passion, impulse and desire, the claims of his ego, domination, power, excitement, battle and struggle, inner and outer adventure.

3. *Mental Man* tends to be subordinate to his mental self-expression, mental aims, mental interests, or to a mental idea or ideal the rest of his being. Philosophers, thinkers, scientist, intellectual creators, idealists and dreamers are put forward as representatives of this type.

None of them represents the final stage, which is represented by the consciousness related to the inner physical, inner vital and inner mental; which is much more comprehensive and powerful. When the subliminal is transcended, the spiritual is born.

4. *Spiritual Man,* efforts of Nature to create "the spiritual sage, seer, prophet, God-lover, yogi, gnostic, sufi, mystic", even after having already evolved "the mental

creator, thinker, sage, prophet of an ideal, the self-controlled, self-disciplined, harmonised human being". (Sri Aurobindo 1970, 1070-1072, Singh 1986, 172-173)

It is worthwhile to note that the two contemporary researchers, having divergent approaches and having never met each other, arrive at identical conclusions, of course, with some differences. Jung is an empirical psychologist, while Sri Aurobindo is a yogi. Jung sees the inadequacy of ego to represent both conscious and the unconscious at the same time, and hence this is the cause of the "division of personality" according to him. He suggests that the ego should be made strong and at the same time it should be made to realised its "subordinate position" to self; and thus both ego and the self should work simultaneously. Sri Aurobindo does not recommend the strengthening of the ego; and, suggests its complete replacement by the psychic being first, and then by the self. Jung considers ego to be the only representative of consciousness, and hence, it is essential for him. However, for Sri Aurobindo, ego is only a stepping stone and obsolete. Self for Jung is only an archetypal representative of the inner reality, and consequently, although it may serve the purpose of integrating the disparate elements of the personality, it has no permanent base or strength to be given to the personality of the individual. On the other hand, "as the self in Sri Aurobindo's system is the absolute merely individualised, it is potent enough to give everything required to the personality, i.e. energy, unity, stability and purpose". (Singh 1986, 175)

Jung advises a duel between the conscious and the unconscious, which, according to him, is the way for the two to reconcile and finally harmonise. Sri Aurobindo's method is to subordinate the outer by the inner and thus get enlightened. Although both want the individual to come out of one's confinement, Jung's individuation does not come unto Sri Aurobindo's purpose to illuminate the lower consciousness by a higher one and get governed by the law of hierarchy. Thus, he wants the people to realise that the physical is under the vital, the vital is under the mental, the outer "physical-vital-mental" is under the internal "physical-vital-mental"; all this grouping is under the psychic, and the psychic is under the spiritual. Jung's individuation envisages a dualism between the objective and the subjective or the matter and the spirit, which may finally churn out some higher principle which is on top of everything. Sri Aurobindo's transformation believes that everything has descended from *Satchidananda*, which is the eternal "higher principle" already in existence. "From this viewpoint, however, the Jungian individuation is a pointer, a stepping stone to the Aurobindonian transformation." (Singh 1986, 177)

Although the two thinkers began and proceeded differently, the convergence of their final results must prove to be the *Confirmation of Truth or Inner Reality,* which should be taken as a goal to be achieved by the people of the world and bring improvement to the society as a whole.

The congruence of their findings can be seen as follows. The predecessors of Jung explained the division of personality by accounting for just one personality, but Jung worked for their integration by a superior and universal personality represented by the self. Similarly, the predecessors of Sri Aurobindo have shown the way of recognising one of the paths only – path of devotion, selfless service or knowledge, etc. – and showing its relevance to the "Supreme Being", but Sri Aurobindo has assigned a proper place to each one of them and has shown the path of transformation and integration of each one with its next higher one, finally leading to a well-balanced personality and recognition of the "Supreme Being". Thus, both the thinkers have worked on the principle of unifying all the factors involved in the process, rather than choosing one and rejecting others. Both individuation and transformation take care of every part of the personality of the individual and aim at unification leading to "wholeness" of the individual. Furthermore, each of them has divided an individual into eight types, showing the congruence in all except the last type of Sri Aurobindo, which belongs to his classification exclusively.

	Jung		*Sri Aurobindo*
i)	Extrovert Sensational	____________	Outer Physical
ii)	Extrovert Feeling	____________	Outer Vital
iii)	Extrovert Thinking	____________	Outer Mental
iv)	Introvert Sensational	____________	Inner Physical
v)	Introvert Feeling	____________	Inner Vital
vi)	Introvert Thinking	____________	Inner Mental
vii)	Intuitive Extrovert / Introvert (both types)	____________	Subliminal Spiritual Type (outside of the scope of Jungian Classification)

One can see that all the eight types of Jung correspond to the first seven types of Sri Aurobindo, while the eighth type of the latter is outside the classification of the former. Another point of difference is that Jung considers his types to be abnormal persons because of the imbalance in different parts of the personality. This is not a happy conclusion, since it means majority of the people on earth are abnormal. Sri Aurobindo, on the other hand, considers his types to be predominated by one aspect as compared to others, on the ladder of evolution. On assimilating each lower aspect into the next higher, one reaches the finale in the spiritual type. This appears to be a better approach.

However, Jung's preference of the introvert over the extrovert is a welcome departure from the usual Western thought which gives preference to an extrovert for success in the physical world. Clearly, introversion is the higher step towards evolution.

Philosophy of Martinus

Another contemporary of Jung and Sri Aurobindo was Martinus of Denmark, born on August 11, 1890 in a small village, Sindal, of Jutland. Martinus was born of an unmarried mother who died when he was a child, and he was raised by his maternal uncle and aunt. He worked in a dairy industry until December 1922, when he left his work in the office of a big Copenhagen dairy in order to devote himself exclusively to the creation of *Livets Bog* (*The Book of Life*). He had no desire to marry and make a home, rather he wanted to go as a missionary to Africa or Eastern countries. His conception of God differed very much from that of the Christian doctrine. According to Erik Gerner Larsson (1963, 10-11), "Martinus borrowed a small theosophical tract from a friend and meditated with his eyes closed by kerchief. After a little while, sitting thus, he suddenly found himself enveloped in a glaring white light, and a number of cosmic experiences took place... The process grew stronger during the following days... He found himself in possession of new senses, enabling him to see not only the world visible to everybody but, besides, all the real causes behind the misery of this world... 'The Great Birth', in the beginning, gave rise to a violent awakening of psychic powers, now generally become latent in most people... After his spiritual experience, it was impossible for him to relish the taste of meat, tobacco and alcoholic beverages." He began writing the *Livets Bog*, the first volume of which was published on the 11th of July, 1932. In November 1932, circles for the study of *Livets Bog* were formed at the Danish towns of Copenhagen, Odense, Arhus and Alborg; and the first issue of the magazine, *Kosmos,* was published on the 1st of April, 1933.

Scandinavian mythology manifests the religious principle in two directly contrary forms: first one impelling the individual to consecrate his life to war so that he, by dying on the "field of honour", should earn the reward of a life of blissfulness in the company of the "gods", whereas the second one for happiness after death relies on charity and unselfishness. The first one is the "dark" from which "dominated humanity, during its slow awakening and unto the time when the three great cosmologic teachers, Buddha, Christ and Mohammed, appeared, and each one separately gave prominence to charity as the only way to a life in perfect happiness... a mode of living directly contrary to the one our ancestors regarded as the only salvation". (Larsson 1963, 27) Martinus described the whole course of evolution from mineral to vegetable to animal kingdom, where we are now.

According to Martinus, "Since everything that is perceptible by the senses such as – solids, gases and cosmic or spiritual substances, or energy, can exist only in the form of vibration or motion, it naturally follows that no absolute 'fixed point' is possible in the material world. However, as everything perceptible or observable is identical with vibration or motion, it is obvious that the fixed point can be only that which perceives the motion. The 'fixed point' in existence, then, is identical with a 'something' capable of perceiving motion. Motion being unable to perceive motion, it must be said 'something' which experiences the motion and not the reverse. It, accordingly, makes its appearance as the master or originator of the motion. Thus, it is recognised that an absolute 'fixed point' exists, around which all vibration or motion takes place; and the fact that this 'fixed point' has experience of the movements makes it the most supreme 'Something' in existence. This supreme 'Something' is 'God Eternal'... The divine presence, or highest 'something' in the living being, is given expression in the concept of 'I'...It has no tangible form, no potential capacity, it only is." (Larsson 1963, 30-33)

This "I" is expressed as "X.1.". Plants have consciousness – this has long been proved by science. Creative impulses are at work even in minerals, although it is difficult to perceive through physical vision. Only cosmic consciousness can perceive that every single atom is creating ceaselessly. This "creative principle" is named as "X.2.". These two eternal varieties would have not been known without the existence of the third one – the Thing Created, called "X.3.". God is the aggregate of the triune principle: the I, the Creative Principle and matter or the Thing Created, that is, "X.1.", "X.2." and "X.3." This analysis, according to Larsson (p.36), holds good for every living being and fully verifies the scriptural text which says that we are created in the "Image of God".

Evolution is a process by which the living being is seen to migrate from the vegetable to animal to the human kingdom and then to the dominion about which Christ said, "My kingdom is not of this world." The third principle of the triune, that is, the Thing Created or matter or energy has six different primary forms. The lowest of them is the Energy of Instinct, as the sustaining factor of consciousness in the vegetable kingdom. The perennial sprouting and blossoming of the "buds", a new flower unfolding the instant its predecessor begins to expire represents the Energy of Instinct. The next is the Energy of Gravity, for example, the Energy of Killing in a carnivorous plant, which comes into existence as "the killing principle" in it wakes to life and takes possession of the consciousness of the plant, urging it on to a new culmination – the animal kingdom. The beautiful petals of its flowers are transformed into teeth and claws, and we now see it as an animal and no longer recognise it as a plant. Thus, a carnivorous plant is at a transitional stage between the vegetable kingdom and animal kingdom. The spirituality is "asleep" at this stage. And then, in the midst of the offending and suffocative situation of "gravity", such as in a war, the third Energy of Feeling takes birth, which seeks disarmament, peace, internationalism, etc. Thus, a longing to resume again the peaceful life it had voluntarily abandoned, begins to grow in its mind. This longing is what we know as religiousness. Thereafter, when the feelings culminate, the energies of intelligence, intuition and memory come forward, in that order. Each energy has its own zone. All these energies are finally comprised in the seventh: the Mother Energy.

The consciousness, and hence, the existence of the individual therefore, passes through the following seven planes, according to the philosophy of Martinus. A comparison with the seven planes of universe drawn in Chapter 1 is also shown in the following table:

S. No.	*Martinus*	*Chapter 1*
1.	Mother Energy	Divine
2.	Memory	Monadic
3.	Intuition	*Atmic*
4.	Intelligence	Intuitional
5.	Feeling	Mental
6.	Gravity	Astral
7.	Instinctive	Physical

4
GATEWAYS TO HIGHER CONSCIOUSNESS

Introduction

Analysis of experiences that are promoted by forces that cannot be sensed by the ordinary physical senses, is called "spiritual knowledge". Human beings are not at the same level in evolution. Just as there are beings who are behind modern science in evolution, so there are also beings who arc "ahead" of it and have already accumulated experiences that are based on spiritual forces. Such people possess "layers of consciousness" which are at present unknown to science and the rest of mankind. These layers of consciousness are called "higher consciousness" by the parapsychologists, "cosmic consciousness" by the transcendentalists and "opening of the third eye" by Vedantists.

What we understand from higher/cosmic consciousness or by consciousness higher than cosmic, has already been defined in the previous chapters. In this chapter, we are concerned with the means of attaining such a consciousness.

The Vedic Method

The goal of human existence is to achieve a state of freedom, in which a cosmic Mind, Life and Matter are acting, or a pure transcendental Self-Power and Bliss other than our own personal being are acting; and this is possible in the following three ways: (i) *Karma yoga* – the "path of selfless action", which requires renunciation of ego, desire and personal initiation and surrender of the being to the cosmic Self or to the universal Power called *Shakti*; (ii) *Jnana yoga* – the "path of knowledge", which requires cessation of thought, silence of mind, opening of the whole being to the cosmic Consciousness or Self or Supreme Reality; (iii) *Bhakti yoga* - the "path of devotion", which requires the surrender of the heart and the whole nature into the hands of All-Blissful as the adored Master of our existence. The culminating transformation unveils the secret Master of our activities gradually, and from the security of the supreme Will and Knowledge, He gives the sanction to the divine *Shakti* of working in us with a purified and exalted manner for her instrument.

The Rishis, experimenting through various methods and knowing the "truth" in their states of *samadhi*, found that the individuals are not at the same physical, mental, emotional and intutitional levels, and consequently, divided human beings into three groups: (i) Rational and intellectuals beings in whom head predominates the heart; (ii) Instinctual and emotional beings in whom heart predominates the head; and (iii) Beings in whom the head and the heart have an almost equal assertion. Accordingly, the methods suitable for them for Self-realisation are: *Jnana yoga* – path of knowledge, *Bhakti yoga* – path of devotion, and *Karma yoga* – path of selfless action, respectively. A fourth category was later designed for those in whom neither the intellectual nor the emotional level was sufficiently developed. A set of rules were originally prescribed and improved gradually over the millenniums. The name given to this kind of yoga is *Hatha yoga,* the greatest exponents of which are known to be the famous saints Patanjali, Gorakh Nath and Jnaneshwar of the medieval ages. *Kundalini yoga* is an improvised form of this yoga and will be dealt with separately.

Out of the four *Vedas,* it is *Yajur Veda* which is devoted to *Karma yoga, Rig Veda* is devoted to *Jnana yoga,* and *Sama Veda* is devoted to *Bhakti yoga.*

In what follows, we shall elaborate on the three basic methods one by one. We shall begin with *Karma yoga* which has received the maximum attention of Lord Krishna in the *Bhagavad Gita* and through which the philosophy of "liberation from falsehood" has been comprehensively explained.

i) *Karma yoga (The Path of Selfless Action)*

Sri Aurobindo (1986, 18-28) has explained *Karma yoga* in a very lucid manner. Present inner life of man which depends mainly on the vital and physical nature is not the whole of real existence. Present nature of man is only an outer appearance of the hidden Self within him. One has to understand the *Sankhya* distinction between the Soul and Nature – the power that knows, supports and informs, and the power that works, acts and provides the different instruments, medium and process. The Soul is immutable omnipresent Self or *Brahman,* while the other soul of Nature is our mutable and dynamic being which deals with the phenomenal world.

Nature acts through three fundamental modes or qualities called *Gunas* – *tamasic, rajasic* and *sattvic.* In *tamasic* action, we have an inert personality which is subject to and satisfied with the mechanical round of things, and is incapable of any strong effort at a freer action or mastery. In *rajasic* action, we have the restless, active personality which forces Nature to serve its needs and desires without really understanding that in doing so it is only fulfilling the demands of Nature itself and, in fact, there is no freedom for us. In *sattvic* action, we try to live as an enlightened personality working on reason and having some preferred ideal or good, truth or beauty; which again is subject to the appearances of Nature and the ideals representing only the changing phases of our personality, which does not lead to a definite rule or any kind of stable satisfaction. Living in any one of the three modes, we only rotate on the wheel of mutation, obeying the Power within, through our ego, and not at all even in communion with that Power, leave alone acting as the Power ourselves. Thus, there is no freedom or mastery but a servitude in fact.

To get freedom, the first thing we have to do is to make our senses free from the grip of external world, that is, to hold back the natural running of our senses after the external objects and to live inwardly. The mastery of senses will bring the realisation of a soul within, which is free from the mutations of mind and is self-existent, tranquil, self-possessed, master of itself and unaffected by the eager running of the outer nature. This can be done by the control on "desire" which seeks to satisfy itself through the senses and whose only occupation is in the play of passions. On destruction of the propensity of our natural being by getting rid of the desire, the passions will fall into quietude, since the joy of possession and grief of loss, success and failure, pleasantness and unpleasantness, which used to entertain the passions, will pass out from the soul. A calmness will then prevail within. Furthermore, since we have yet to live in the world and work, and our nature has been to seek the fruits of our works, we must bring a radical change in our nature to work, but without attachment to the fruits of the works. This will eradicate desire and its results. And this change in nature of the doer can be brought about by dissociating works from ego and personality, through the reasoning that this is only the play of the *Gunas* of Nature. This understanding will dissociate the soul from the play by becoming the "observer" of the workings of Nature and leaving those works to the Power behind which is the Master of the universe, which is greater than ourselves. The only obstacle in getting this done is the "mind", whose nature is to run after the senses along with its reason and will. This brings us to learn to still the mind, which leads to the awareness of the self, which is calm, motionless and blissful, untroubled and unaffected by the outer things of the world, self-sufficient and living in eternal satisfaction.

Karma yoga, therefore, requires the perfection of the being in the following steps:

1. Consecrate all our works as a sacrifice to the Divine in us and in the world. It is not difficult to initiate such an attitude of the mind and heart, but it is also not easy to remain sincere and all-pervasive in our efforts.
2. Renounce attachment to the fruits of our works. The only desirable fruit is the Divine Presence, Consciousness and power in us. If this is achieved, everything else will be added. This is the transformation of the egoistic will, desire-soul and desire-nature. Naturally, the second step is more difficult than the first.
3. Get rid of the central egoism, the sense of being the worker or doer. The third step is yet more difficult than the first two. However, as soon as the ego-sense

is rooted out from the nature, one knows one's true person which stands out as a part of the Divine and one can renounce everything other than the will of the Divine Power or *Shakti*.

4. Give up the proprietorship of all material possessions. When the self is revealed within us and we begin to feel its peace and stillness, we can grow into that and carry things to their fullness – calm, equal, passionless, impersonal, all-pervading self. Senses become still, ego dissolves into impersonal existence; our works cease to be ours, cease to bind or trouble us; Nature and her *Gunas* continue to work, but without affecting our griefless self-existent tranquillity. All is given up into that one equal and universal *Brahman*. (Sri Aurobindo 1986, 327)

"Once free, he has only to continue working in the sphere assigned to him by Fate and circumstances till the great hour arrives when he can at last disappear into the Infinite." (Sri Aurobindo 1986, 211)

ii) *Jnana yoga*

The "path of knowledge" is perhaps in prominence at present since it includes the "official science", which is in search of "truth" in its own experimental way; and the "western approach", which is mainly the intellectual search for "truth". This also includes the parapsychological and psychic search, for example, the work of Jung and others. Yet, the recognition of potentialities of human intellect by *Vedanta* will leave the people stand aghast at their own incapacity to make complete use of their intellect in search of "truth". *Vedanta* travels the path of pure reason and inculcates in us the "jewel of discrimination" between the false and true in us; between the permanent and temporal; between the real and unreal; and leads us to self-discovery, to the knowledge that Self and God are one by identity.

This is the glory of Hinduism. The path has also been called *Raja yoga,* meaning, the king of yogas. King Janaka, father-in-law of Lord Rama, was perhaps the first recognised "raja yogi".

Ramana Maharshi used to think all the time of only one thing – who am I? And one day, he arrived at the realisation that *atman* and *Brahman* are identical. Shankaracharya, Vivekananda, Socrates, Aristotle, Plato, Gurdjief, Steiner, William Wordsworth, Richard Maurice Bucke, etc. were all thinkers belonging to the category of a "raja yogi", of course, there may be variations in their stages of perfection. The progression of steps is more or less the same as in *Karma yoga,* and of course, the final realisation too is the same. One goes on removing cover after cover of ignorance, just like removing the sheaths of a cabbage or onion one by one, and finally reaches the goal one day. Beginning with the *Vedanta,* a vast literature is available, both in the East and the West. For example, Swami Vivekananda has written fifteen volumes of nearly five hundred pages each on the subject.

The fact is that the knowledge takes the individual to a certain stage of development or evolution; and then, the mind ceases to exist and wisdom takes over, which is a direct perception of truth from beyond. The following observations should prove enlightening. We begin with Sri Aurobindo (1982, 3-35):

"Late, I learned that when reason died, the Wisdom was born; before that liberation, I had only knowledge."

"There are two allied powers in man: knowledge and wisdom. Knowledge is so much of the truth, seen in a distorted medium, as the mind arrives at groping; wisdom, what the eye of divine vision sees in the spirit."

"When I speak, the reason says, This will I say; but God takes the word of my mouth and the lips say something else, at which reason trembles."

"If mankind could see, though in a glimpse of fleeting experience, what infinite enjoyments, what perfect forces, what luminous reaches of spontaneous knowledge, what wide calms of our being lie waiting for using the tracts which our animal evolution has not yet conquered, they would leave all and never rest till they had gained these treasures. But the way is narrow, the doors are hard to force, and fear, distrust and scepticism are there, sentinels of Nature, to forbid the turning away of our feet from her ordinary pastures."

"Reason divides, fixes details and contrasts them; Wisdom unifies, marries contrasts in a single harmony."

"What the soul sees and has experienced, that it knows; the rest is appearance, prejudice and opinion."

"Immortality is not the survival of the mental personality after death, though that also is true, but the waking possession of the unborn and deathless Self, of which body is only an instrument and a shadow."

"They proved to me by convincing reasons that God did not exist, and I believed them. Afterwards I saw God, for He came and embraced me. And now which I am to believe, the reasoning of others or my own experience?"

"Hallucination is the term of Science for those irregular glimpses we still have, of truths shut out from us by our preoccupation with matter... That which men term a hallucination is the reflection in the mind and senses of that which is beyond our ordinary mental and sensory perceptions."

"Logic is the worst enemy of Truth, as self-righteousness is the worst enemy of virtue; for the one cannot see its own errors nor the other its own imperfections."

"The sign of dawning Knowledge is to feel that as yet I know little or nothing; and yet, if I could only know my knowledge, I already possess everything."

"When Wisdom comes, her first lesson is, 'There is no such thing as knowledge; there are only apercus of the Infinite Deity.'"

"If men took life less seriously, they could very soon make it more perfect. God never takes his works seriously; therefore one looks out on this wonderful Universe."

"The supernatural is that the nature of which we have not yet attained or do not yet know, or the means of which we have not yet conquered. The common taste for miracles is the sign that man's ascent is not yet finished."

"Pain is the touch of our Mother teaching us how to bear and grow in rapture. She has three stages of her schooling, endurance first, next equality of soul, last ecstasy."

"Only by perfect renunciation of desire or by perfect satisfaction of desire can the utter embrace of God be experienced, for in both ways, the essential precondition is effected – the desire perishes."

"Revelation is the direct sight, the direct hearing or the inspired memory of Truth, *dristi, sruti, smriti;* it is the highest experience and always accessible to renewed experience. Not because God spoke it, but because the soul saw it, is the word of the Scriptures our supreme authority."

"*Sannyas* (renunciation) has a formal garb and outer tokens; therefore, men think they can easily recognise it; but the freedom of Janaka (father-in-law of Lord Rama) does not proclaim itself and it wears the garb of the world; to its presence, even Narada (great sage) was blinded... Unless thou canst see the soul, how shalt thou say that a man is free or bound?"

"Knowledge is a child with its achievements, it runs about the streets whooping and shouting; Wisdom conceals hers for a long time in a thoughtful and mighty silence."

"The love of solitude is a sign of the disposition towards knowledge; but the knowledge itself is only achieved when we have a settled perception of solitude in the crowd, in the battle and in the mart."

"If when thou art doing great actions and moving giant results, thou canst perceive that *thou* art doing nothing, then know that God has removed His seal from thy eyelids."

"All disease is a means towards some new joy of health, all evil and pain a tuning of Nature for some more intense bliss and good, all death an opening of widest immortality. Why and how this should be so is God's secret, which only the soul purified of egoism can penetrate."

"There are two for whom there is hope, the man who has felt God's touch and been drawn to it and the sceptical seeker and self-convinced atheist; but for the formularists of all the religions and the parrots of free thoughts, they are dead souls, who follow a death that they call living."

"What was Ramakrishna? God manifest in a human being; but behind there is God in His infinite personality and His universal personality. And what was Vivekananda? A radiant glance from the eye of Shiva; but behind him is the divine gaze from which he came and Shiva himself and Brahma and Vishnu and Om all-exceeding."

"The double law of sin and virtue is imposed on us because we have not that ideal life and knowledge within which guides the soul spontaneously and infallibly to its self-fulfilment. The law of sin and virtue ceases for us when the sun of God shines upon the soul in truth and love with its unveiled splendour. Moses is replaced by Christ, the *Shastra* by the *Veda*."

"Christ came into the world to purify, not to fulfil. He himself foreknew the failure of his mission and the necessity of his return with the sword of God into a world that had rejected him."

"Mohammed's mission was necessary, else we might have ended by thinking, in the exaggeration of our efforts at self-purification, that earth was meant only for the monk and the city created as a vestibule for the desert."

"Law cannot save the world, therefore Moses' ordinances are dead for humanity and the *Shastra* of the Brahmins is corrupt and dying. Law released into freedom is the liberator. Not the Pundit, but the Yogi; not monasticism, but the inner renunciation of desire and ignorance and egoism."

"In God's providence there is no evil; but only good or its preparation."

"Live within; be not shaken by outward happenings."

"Ancient India, with its ideal of vast riches and vast spendings, was the greatest of nations. Modern India, with its trend towards national asceticism, has fully become poor in life and sunk into weakness and degradation."

"Religion and philosophy seek to rescue man from his ego; then the kingdom of heaven within will be spontaneously reflected in an external divine city."

"Vedanta says rather, 'Man, thou art of one nature and substance with God, one soul with thy fellow-men. Awake and progress then to the utter divinity, live for God in thyself and in others.' This gospel which was given only to the few, must now be offered to all mankind for its deliverance."

In what follows, we present the quotations from various saints which confirm the identity of soul with God:

"Why should man go about seeking God? He is in the heart-beats and thou knowest it not; thou went in error in seeking Him outside thyself."

"God is my inmost self, the reality of my being."

— *Vivekananda*

"He who finds not the Eternal in himself, will never find it outside; but he who sees Him in the temple of his own soul, sees Him also in the temple of the universe."

"The individual I' and the supreme Spirit are one and the same. The difference lies in degree: the one is finite, the other infinite; the one is dependent, the other independent."

— *Ramakrishna*

"Where should thou seek God? Seek Him in thy soul which is eternal in its nature and contains the divine birth."

— *Boehme*

"Heaven is within thee. If thou seek God elsewhere, thou wilt never find Him."

"Thou should not cry after God: the source is in thyself."

"I know that I have in me something without which nothing could be. It is that I call God."

— *Angelus Silesius*

"God cannot be recognised except in oneself. So long as thou findest Him not in thee, thou wilt not find Him anywhere. There is no God for the man who does not find Him in himself."

"The greatest joy man can conceive is the joy of recognising in himself a being free, intelligent, loving and in consequence happy, of feeling God in himself."

"Man, in order to be really a man, must conceive the idea of God in himself."

— Tolstoy

"While thou art saying 'I am alone with myself', in thy heart there is dwelling uninterruptedly that supreme Spirit, silent observer of all good and all evil."

— Laws of Manu

"Thou seest Him, yet thou knowest not that thou seest."
"Thou are not, but only He."
"Thou art He and He is thou."
"All the attributes of Allah are thy attributes."

— Mohyuddin Ibn Arabi

"The supreme Brahman, the self of all, the great abode of the universe, more subtle than the subtle, eternal, That is thyself and thou art That."

— Kaivalya Upanishad

"Thou art That... not a part, not a mode of It, but identically That, the absolute Spirit."

— Chandogya Upanishad

"The essence of our being, the mystery in us which calls itself 'I' – what words have we to express things like these? It is breath of Heaven; the Highest reveals itself in man. This body, these faculties, this life that we live, is it not all a robe for Him who is nameless?"

— Carlyle

"God is myself; we are one in consciousness and His knowing is my knowing."
"If I were not, God would not be."

— Eckhart

"The Purusha who is there and there, He am I."

— *Isha Upanishad*

"They regarded the divine Being and grew assured that it was no other than themselves... that they were themselves that Being... that they and that Being made but one."

— *Fariduddin Attar*

The above quotes are taken from *The Eternal Wisdom.* (Sri Aurobindo Ashram, Pondicherry, 1993)

iii) *Bhakti yoga (The Path of Devotion)*

Out of the four *Vedas,* it is *Sama Veda* which deals with *bhakti* (devotion) and Lord Krishna categorically declared to Arjuna that amongst all the *Vedas,* it is the *Sama Veda* which he considers to be most important. In His own words, "Of the Vedas, I am the Sama Veda..." (*Bhagavad Gita* 10: 22) The paths of selfless action and knowledge bring the individual to the realisation that the self or *atman* is identical with *Brahman.* "But, it is dry knowledge; it is *rasa* (joy) and *rasa* alone which surrounds it (*bhakti*) on all sides and permeates it. God Himself is *rasa* personified and it is *rasa* which is the abode of supreme bliss. It is through *bhakti* alone that one can perceive God, the embodiment of *rasa.*" (Poddar n.d. Preface, ix) According to Poddar, practice of *bhakti* is the foremost discipline for the attainment of Divine Love, and as an end it is this *bhakti* which manifests itself as Divine Love. The secret of the Beloved can be known only through intimate, exclusive, constant and unalloyed love. In the words of Dr. Chaturbhuj Sahai, "In the close proximity of God, when the love-intoxicated practitioner begins to get absorbed in His consciousness, then this is called 'upasana', the deeper state of which is called 'samadhi'. Yoga or meeting is possible only in *samadhi.*" (Sahai 1990, 16)

According to Sahai, some people try to get absorbed in the consciousness of God by attaining detachment. But deep breathing and other metaphysical practices are not enough; they can bring detachment, of course, but you need something more than that.

Although one can, and there have been innumerable people who directly plunged into the path of *bhakti* or devotion, the better and more rewarding way is through selfless action (*karma*) and knowledge (*jnana*). *Bhakti* is not opposed to *karma,* and there is no antagonism between *jnana* and *bhakti.* In fact, those alone who possess real wisdom and knowledge of Truth are really qualified to obtain Divine Love. Poddar has written a commentary on the aphorisms of Devarsi Narada, which is devoted to the exposition of *bhakti* as directed towards a Personal God, discussed the hindrances to the growth of *bhakti,* the means of attaining *bhakti* and the glory of *bhakti* and the *bhakts.* Even Lord Krishna has stated in the *Bhagavad Gita* that a devotee who is knowledgeable and wise, is specially loving to Him.

Maharshi Vyas was in possession of the spiritual vision; he divided the *Vedas* into four parts, composed the *Mahabharata* and called it the fifth *Veda,* brought forth the *Puranas,* and yet he had not peace in his heart, as if something was still missing. Devarshi Narada, then, appeared before him and told him that the reason for his unhappiness was that he had not sung the praises of God and had not described the glories of God to the extent that he had described other aspects of *Dharma*. Devarshi Narada, who knew the truths of the *Vedas,* placed *bhakti* (devotion) at a very high place. In *Bhakti-Rasayana,* Madhusudan Saraswati has divided *bhakti* into elevent stages: (1) Personal service of *Mahapurusha* (great men).

(2) Acquiring of qualifications so as to draw their compassion. (3) Faith in the *Dharma* practised by them. (4) Hearing the Divine glory with reverence. (5) From hearing, growth of the germ of Divine Love. (6) Divine Love leading to Self-realisation. (7) Self-realisation leading to increase of Love in the supreme embodiment of Bliss. (8) Through increase of Love, germination of supreme Bliss. (9) Firm adherence to *Bhagavata Dharma.* (10) Development of the qualities of a *bhagavata* within the devotee. (11) Attainment of the highest stage of Love.

According to *Bhakti Sutras* of Devarshi Narada, *bhakti* or devotion is the development of *exclusive Love* for God, which is nectarean in character; and its attainment gives perfection, immortality and thorough satisfaction. On attainment of *Love,* one stops craving for anything, stops grieving over any loss, neither hates nor delights in any object, nor does he feel any urge for the acquisition of sense-objects; one becomes mad, silent and delighted in self. *Love* has no element of desire in it, being of the nature of *nirodha* (renunciation). Renuciation consists in relinquishing all forms of action, secular as well as religious; it may also be called an exclusive feeling towards God and indifference to everything hostile to God. In exclusiveness, one gives up dependence on everything else except on the Beloved Lord. Indifference to all that is antagonistic to God consists in conforming one's activities, both secular and religious, to the will of God. One should scrupulously respect the injunctions of the scriptures, otherwise there is a risk of fall. There is a stage when all activities, religious as well as mundane, drop off as a matter of course; but until that stage is reached, both these forms of duty should be scrupulously performed.

Different schools have different definitions of *bhakti* (love). According to Maharishi Vedavyasa, son of Parasara, *bhakti* means attachment to the worship of God and other allied practices. In the opening of Garga, *bhakti* means fondness for hearing the stories of the various sports of the Lord. In view of Sandilya, it is supreme attachment to God, which is not opposed to love of self. Devarshi Narada sums up all these definitions and says that *bhakti* consists in offering all activities to God and in feeling immensely restless and miserable at the slightest lapse in the remembrance of God. Lord Krishna has declared in the *Bhagavad Gita* that amongst all types of Yogis, one who adoreth Him with reverence and with his inner-self abiding in Him, is considered to be the best by Him. (6: 47) Narada has given examples of the devotion of *gopis* (milkmaids), who are already in eternal union with the Lord, and they do not need any kind of yoga or meditation for the same. Even in the state of forgetfulness, there is no absence of the Divine glory in the *gopis.* Love which is bereft of this knowledge of Divine Glory, is of the category of the love of a paramour, in which, there is no deriving of joy from the beloved.

According to Narada (*Bhakti Sutra 25*), Divine Love is superior even to *karma* (action), *jnana* (knowledge) and yoga; it is an end in itself. Even God has aversion for pride and loves humility. Some thinkers are of the opinion that *jnana* (knowledge) is the only means of attaining Love or Devotion. According to some others, *bhakti* and *jnana* are interdependent. According to Narada and other sons of Brahma, *bhakti* is an end in itself; and hence, the seekers of liberation must adopt the path of devotion.

Coming to the methods of devotion, the teachers and prophets have prescribed renunciation of worldly objects and worldly attachments. Success is attained through ceaseless *bhajans* (religious songs in the glory of Lord). But the primary means are said to be the grace of a *Mahapurusha* (Great Soul, who has realised God) or an iota of Divine grace; after which, other practices follow as a matter of course. However, contact with a *Mahapurusha* is rare, it becomes possible through His grace. Since there is no difference between God and His devotee, it is therefore recommended that one should cultivate contact with a Lover of God.

Evil company is said to be the main obstacle to Divine Love, since such a company breeds lust, anger, infatuation, loss of memory, loss of wisdom and total ruin, which appear in the form of ripples in the beginning and assume the dimensions of an ocean later.

One who renounces all attachments, who serves great souls and who does not regard anything as one's own, is the one who crosses *maya* (illusion). One who lives in seclusion, snaps all ties with the world, transcends the three *gunas* (modes of nature) and gives up all thoughts of *yog* (providing the needs) and *kshem* (safety of one's possessions). One who renounces not only the fruit of action but the action itself, and thus renouncing everything, becomes indifferent to all pairs of opposites. One who totally renounces even the *Vedas* and who attains ceaseless, unbounded Love of God, is the one who crosses *maya* (illusion) and guides others across the *maya.*

Divine Love cannot be described in words; it is like the pleasure of the palate enjoyed by a dumb person. One who is in it does not speak, and one who speaks is not in it. It manifests itself in rare persons who are qualified for it. This Love has no qualities and has no desires, every moment it increases from more to more, it is subtler than the subtlest and it is of the nature of experience. On attaining this Love, the devotee sees nothing but Love, hears only about Love, speaks only of Love and thinks only of Love. Divine Love being considered primary, the secondary Love or Devotion is of three kinds, according to three *Gunas* or Modes of Nature: *Sattvic* (pure), *Rajasic* (active) and *Tamasic* (having inertia), as defined earlier with greater details.

According to Narada, amongst all forms of spiritual practices the practice of Devotion is the easiest, which is a proof in itself. It is of the nature of Peace and Supreme Bliss.

After surrendering oneself and one's interests (temporal and spiritual) to God, the practitioner should not worry about the worldly losses. However, worldly activities should not be abandoned until one reaches perfection in devotion and one should practise devotion in a disinterested way, renouncing the fruit of action. One should not hear the talks about women, wealth, unbelievers and enemies. One should avoid pride, hypocrisy, etc. Having offered all activities to God, if the practitioner is still haunted by lust, anger, pride, etc., these should be directed towards God Himself. Making God the object of one's passion, anger, pride, etc., would then be the best way to get rid of them.

One should dissolve the triple consciousness (worship, worshipper and the object of worship) and cultivate Love alone in the form of incessant service of the Lord of incessant wifely devotion to the Lord. Supreme Devotion to the Lord is even superior to five types of *mukti* or liberation (Poddar n.d. 185): (i) *Salokya* (residence in the abode of the Lord), (ii) *Samipya* (living in close proximity to the Lord), (iii) *Sarsti* (enjoying the same powers as the Lord), (iv) *Saripya* (having a similar form to that of the Lord) and (v) *Sayujya* (absolute identity with the Lord).

Devotees who are exclusively attached to the Lord are the best amongst all. Such devotees, conversing with each other in an emotionally choked voice, hair on the body bristling with joy and eyes wet with tears, sanctify their race and earth too. They enhance the sanctity of sacred places, add glory to actions and lend authorities to scriptures because they are one with the Lord. When such a devotee comes into being, his ancestors in heaven or other worlds rejoice, celestial beings dance with joy and the earth finds a protector in him. Among the devotees, there is no distinction due to caste, learning, external appearance, birth, possessions, occupation, etc., since they all belong to Him. To discriminate amongst the devotees is an offence; however, there are said to be sixty-four kinds of offences in general. (See for example, the listing in Poddar n.d. 197-199)

One should never enter into a controversy because there is a chance of excessiveness in arguments and one may not be able to arrive at any conclusion. One should meditate upon the teachings of scriptures which promote devotion and one should perform actions which may be an aid to devotion. According to Poddar (pp.208-209), the following ten principles constitute the principal forms of activities which aid the attainment of Divine Love:

1. Scrupulous observance of duties prescribed for one's *Varna* and *Ashram*. Renunciatory conduct on the part of the *Brahmachari*, Vanaprasthi and *Sanyasi*, and on the part of the *Grahastha* (householder), maintenance of parents, wife, children and other dependants with proper respect and affection in the spirit of thereby earning the pleasure of God, earning of livelihood through truthful and righteous means and performance of sacrifices, charity and austerities, enjoined by the scriptures.

2. Practice of *Sadachara* (right conduct).
3. Attendance in *Satsanga* and hearing and *Kirtan* of Divine Glory and meditation on the same.
4. Practice of *Japa* of the Divine Name, and remembrance and *Kirtan* (loud chanting) of the same.
5. Worship of God, prayer and obeisance.
6. Personal service of saints and devotees and carrying out their behests with reverence.
7. Residence in places of pilgrimage.
8. Compassion for distressed creatures and their service to the best of one's ability through body, mind and wealth.
9. Offering of all actions to God.
10. The practice of observing God in every creature.

Lord Krishna describes in the *Bhagavad Gita* the marks of the loving devotees who are dear to Him as follows (Prabhupad 1989):

"One who is not envious but is a kind friend to all living entities, who does not think himself a proprietor and is free form false ego, who is equal in both happiness and distress, who is tolerant, always satisfied, self-controlled, and engaged in devotional service with determination, his mind and intelligence fixed on Me – such a devotee of mine is very dear to Me." (12: 13-14)

"He for whom no one is put into difficulty and who is not disturbed by anyone, who is equipoised in happiness and distress, fear and anxiety, is very dear to Me." (12: 15)

"My devotee who is not dependent on the ordinary course of activities, who is pure, expert, without cares, free from all pains, and not striving for some results, is very dear to Me." (12: 16)

"One who neither rejoices nor grieves, who neither laments nor desires, and who renounces both auspicious and inauspicious things – such a devotee is very dear to Me." (12: 17)

"One who is equal to friends and enemies, who is equipoised in honour and dishonour, heat and cold, happiness and distress, fame and infamy, who is always free form contaminating association, always silent and satisfied with anything, who does not care for any residence, who is fixed in knowledge and who is engaged in devotional service – such a person is very dear to Me." (12: 18-19)

"Those who follow this imperishable path of devotional service and who completely engage themselves with faith, making Me the supreme goal, are very, very dear to Me." (12: 20)

A God-realised person should be in possession of these marks.

One should not waste even half a second without *bhajan* (repeating the name of God) in awaiting the auspicious moment when one would be free from pleasure and pain, desire and sense of worldly gain, since attention should be on perfection of means and not the end, which is bound to follow if the means are perfected and may slip off otherwise. Every single breath should be as carefully devoted to the remembrance of God as a miser uses his limited number of coins. One should scrupulously observe all aspects of *sadachara* (right conduct) like *ahimsa* (non-injury to others), truth, purity (external and internal), compassion, faith in the existence of God, etc. A God-realised person cannot be judged from the external conduct, nevertheless, there are certain qualities which are bound to be present in him, such as those mentioned above.

When chanting is done with love, God speedily reveals Himself and blesses the practitioner with His perception.

Saints, men of wisdom, the *Puranas* and the *Vedas,* all declare that there is no difference between *Saguna* (Divine manifestation of God with attributes) and *Aguna* (the Absolute). He who is Absolute, Formless, Invisible, Unborn appears as *Saguna* (with attributes) compelled by the Love of the devotee. "That form of God is not a creation of *Maya.* It is wholly a Divine and Supernatural Form; drawn by the Love of the devotee when it manifests itself before him, it makes itself perceptible by raising the devotee to the divine level." (Poddar n.d. 247)

According to Devarshi Narada, amongst all the three forms of Truth practised through the body, speech and mind, the path of *bhakti* is the best, which he repeatedly declares. His statement is corroborated by the *Tripadibhutinarayana-Upanishad,* in the following words, "Abandoning all other methods, take recourse only to *Bhakti.* Be devoted to *Bhakti,* be devoted only to *Bhakti.* Through *Bhakti* all forms of perfection are easily attained. There is nothing which cannot be attained by *Bhakti.*" Other disciplines bring realisation of God in other forms, but through the path of devotion, He is realised as the Beloved.

Although enough has been said about *bhakti* or devotion, yet I cannot hold myself back from citing the quotes by Sri Aurobindo (1982, 72-93), which reveal the Truth of highest order. Out of many, I have selected a few as follows:

"Canst thou see God as the bodiless Infinite and yet love Him as a man loves his mistress? Then has the highest truth of the infinite revealed to thee. Canst thou also clothe the Infinite in one secret embraceable body and see Him seated in each and all of these bodies that are visible and sensible? Then has its widest and profoundest truth come also into the possession."

"To the soul that has hold of the highest beatitude, life cannot be an evil or a sorrowful illusion; rather all life becomes the rippling love and laughter of a divine Lover and Playfellow."

"After I knew that God was a woman, I learned something from far about love; but it was only when I became a woman and served my Master and Paramour that I knew love utterly."

"To commit adultery with God is the perfect experience for which the world was created."

"The Jew invented the God-fearing man; India, the God-knower and God-lover."

"The servant of God was born in Judae, but he came to maturity among the Arabs. India's joy is in the servant-lover."

"If you cannot make God love you, make Him fight you. If He will not give you the embrace of the lover, compel Him to give you the embrace of the wrestler. My soul is the captive of God, taken by Him in battle; it still remembers the war, though so far from it, with delight and alarm and wonder."

"There are three stages in the pain that God gives to us; when it is only pain; when it is pain that causes pleasure; and when it is purely a fiercer form of delight."

"Even when one has climbed up into those levels of bliss where pain vanishes, it still survives disguised as intolerable ecstasy."

"When I was mounting upon ever higher crests of His joy, I asked myself whether there was no limit to the increase of bliss and almost I grew afraid of God's embraces."

"For monogamy may be the best for body, but the soul that loves God in men dwells here always as the boundless and ecstatic polygamist; yet all the time – that is the secret – it is in love with only one being."

"What is the use of admiring Nature or worshipping her as a power, a Presence and a goddess? What is the use, either, of appreciating her aesthetically or artistically? The secret is to enjoy her with the soul as one enjoys a woman with the body."

"The *Mayavadin* talks of my personal God as a dream and prefers to dream of Impersonal Being; the Buddhist puts that aside too as a fiction and prefers to dream of *Nirvana* and the bliss of nothingness. Thus, all the dreamers are busy reviling each other's visions and parading their own as the panacea. What the soul utterly rejoices in, is for thought the ultimate reality."

"Beyond Personality, the *Mayavadin* sees indefinable Existence; I followed him there and found my Krishna beyond in indefinable Personality."

"God has so arranged life that the worked is the soul's husband; Krishna its divine paramour. We owe a debt of service to the world and are bound to it by a law, a compelling opinion, and a common experience of pain and pleasure, but our heart's worship and our free and secret joy are for our Lover."

"The joy of God is secret and wonderful; it is a mystery and a rapture at which common sense makes mouths of mockery; but the soul that has once tasted it, can never renounce, whatever the worldly disrepute, torture and affliction it may bring us."

"The sceptic mind doubts always because it cannot understand, but the faith of the God-lover persists in knowing although it cannot understand. Both are necessary to our darkness, but there can be no doubt which is the mightier. What I cannot understand now, I shall some day master, but if I lose faith and love, I fall utterly from the goal which God has set before me."

Dr. Chaturbhuj Sahai, a realised person himself, went personally into the city where the great saint Mira Bai lived some four to five hundred years ago. Saint Mira Bai used to talk to and live with God Personified for hours and days altogether. In what follows, findings of Sahai (1990) are described briefly.

"*Bhakti* (devotion), *Jnana* (knowledge) and Yoga are stairs leading to Love. Love comes after all these disciplines and as soon as it comes, it bathes the person with bliss. With the invent of Love, virtues such as lustlessness, egolessness, giving up of material possessions and renunication, etc., enter the heart. The moment one dives in the ocean of Love, God appears before the individual. Love has such a power of attraction that it not only draws near the human beings, but even God is drawn close to the devotee. However, Love makes the person appear strange, one loses one's consciousness too. One forgets eating, drinking, sleeping, waking, etc. Turmoil of separation from the Beloved makes one suffer in inner agitation. Home, family, relatives, everyone is left out. Joy or grief, profit or loss, all such thoughts run away. Such is the glory of Love. When the practitioner reaches the highest summit of bliss, Love comes into being at that time. Faith and devotion are lower stages compared to the stage of Love. It is impossible for a normal person to visualise the situation in which a Love-intoxicated person meets the personalised form of God, nevertheless, there are a large number of true life cases in which this has happened. An outstanding case is that of Saint Mira Bai."

There was a scuffle for a statue of Sri Krishna between Mira, who was ten years old then, and a *sadhu* (religious devotee) perhaps in his sixties. The matter went to the king and even he could not resolve it, since both the persons very strongly wanted to possess the statue which belonged to the *sadhu.* For seven days, Mira was crying. Her Love forced God to appear before her. Mira suddenly felt somewhat sleepy and she entered the state of dreaming; she saw a "strange loving being" standing before her who said, "Mira! One whom you have been remembering for the last seven days is 'myself', present before you. Seeing your Love, I have forgotten everything. Tell me whatever you want." To Mira, this was the first *darshan* (seeing in person) of the Lord. There was no limit to her joy. Although she could hardly speak anything, she said in most loving voice, "Lord! Who are you? Are you the same Girdharlalji (a name of Lord Krishna) who is asking me? If you are really pleased with me, then I do not want anything except Yourself and Your Love. If you accept this, then give it to me." Saying these things her throat became dry, tears began to flow from her eyes, and she was wonderstruck for a while. Seeing her in such a condition, Lord held her to His bosom and in a very loving voice He said, "Mira! Do not become sad. You are very loving to me, I belong to you. Whenever you want you will see me before yourself. If there is something in the world that I like, it is one and the only Love. Wherever a devotee remembers me, I go there. Although I am close to everyone, yet the devotees recognise me and consequently they derive bliss from me and even I enjoy the happiness with them."

And, at the same time, the Lord approached the sadhu in another form. While the *sadhu* was fast asleep, he suddenly heard very loud words, "You give my statue to Mira. I am highly pleased with her." The *sadhu* was astonished. He was not sure about what had happened. Just then, he heard again, "You give my statue to Mira, I want to live with her only." Now the eyes of the *sadhu* were opened. He could understand that that small girl was some "high soul". He immediately ran to the palace, surrendered the statue to the king to be passed on to Mira. Mira began to worship the Lord through that statue in various forms, sometimes she would sing songs to Him, sometimes she would dance before Him. The point to be noted here is that the Lord appeared before the *sadhu* only in the form of a voice to give him instructions; while He appeared in full human form before Mira and talked to her in a very loving way. That is, the appearance of the Lord before a devotee is proportional to one's intensity of devotion.

Later in life, even after her marriage, Mira continued to love Sri Krishna. Her husband, the king, deposed her to a ghostly and abandoned palace without the services of any servant or helper. The king thought she would now forget Krishna and come to her senses. After a few months, on visiting her place, he found that the abandoned palace was converted into a well-decorated palace and all things of comfort were there. It was known that Lord Krishna used to be with his beloved Mira for several hours every day in full physical form and both of them used to enjoy all heights of love with each other. According to Mira, she had married Krishna in her dream long back and He only was her husband, no one else. Mira now looked more happy, healthy and satisfied.

Saint Mira Bai is supposed to have existed in A.D. fifteenth century, although there is some uncertainty about it. Nature or the divine plan pushed her to circumstances one after another which led to love of God. She lost her mother in early childhood, got the statue of God at the age of ten, met with a realised saint, separation from husband, meeting with Guru Raidasji who initiated her, the king's disbelief of her and his ill-treatment with her, and so on. Every happening pushed her further towards God and obstacles became the ways and means of achievements. It was all the grace of God. Long back in time, devotees like Prahalad and Dhruv existed, whom every Hindu remembers with great reverence. Like Mira, these two devotees loved God from early childhood and God manifested several times before them. Ramakrishna Paramahansa used to talk to the Lord everyday. Well-known Swami Vivekananda saw and talked with Mother Goddess in her full physical form. Child Namdev, with his intense love, compelled God to materialise before him in physical form and eat food with him. Sri Aurobindo experienced the presence of Mother Goddess as well as Lord Krishna, of which he has talked so confidently in his writings.

Lastly, I can briefly state my own experiences with God Absolute, which have been described in detail in my previous book (Kumar 1998). During the period of meditation, I saw Mother Goddess materialise before me and she moved her hand on my head for her blessings. This happened with me at least three times in a period of six months. Child Brahman materialised before me in the twilight period twice in the month of January 1988, while I was in England. I experienced myself as a "dimensionless being" on some spiritual planet several times. I experienced the "divine female kiss" on my lips in Delhi in the moments of loneliness, which kept me blissfully happy for almost the whole day. My involvement with the world, for example, in writing books or lecturing around and meeting friends and relatives, is keeping me away from more profound experiences. Although I resigned from the position of professor of mathematics in 1994, I have not yet gone into total renunciation. Even the statement of experiences as here may not be justified in the real religious framework. But then how do I confirm with the findings of others to say for sure that God, who is the ocean of love and mercy, does materialise before you, of course, proportional to the intensity of Love?

Summary of Vedic Method: In the words of Lord Krishna, according to *Bhagavad Gita* (Prabhupad 1989):

"Just fix your mind upon Me, the Supreme Personality of Godhead, and engage all your intelligence in Me. Thus you will live in Me always, without doubt. (12: 8)

"If you cannot fix your mind upon Me without deviation, then follow the regulative principle of *bhakti-yoga.* In this way, develop a desire to attain Me." (12: 9)

"If you cannot practice the regulations of *bhakti-yoga,* then just try to work for Me, because by working for Me you will come to the perfect stage." (12: 10)

"If, however, you are unable to work in this consciousness of Me, then try to act giving up all results of your work and try to be self-situated." (12: 11)

"If you cannot take to this practice, then engage yourself in the cultivation of knowledge. Better than knowledge, however, is meditation, and better than meditation is renunciation of the fruits of action, for by such renunciation one can attain peace of mind." (12: 12)

In very clear words, the methods of attaining God-realisation have been described, according to the order of their effectiveness. If one cannot fix one's attention directly on Krishna (or the alternative representation of God, such as Rama, Shiva, Vishnu, etc., as explained by Lord Krishna himself in a separate verse), then the principles of *bhakti-yoga* are recommended, failing which one should begin with the renunciation of the fruits of action which will bring one to the stage of knowledge. Knowledge will gradually bring one to the point of meditation, and meditation will gradually make one know the Supreme Personality of Godhead. Thus, there are two processes; an indirect one as described in this paragraph (*Karma yoga - Jnana yoga - Ashtanga yoga - Bhakti yoga,* beginning with the first and ending with the last, in this order) and a direct one which is the path of devotion, called *Bhakti yoga.*

Comments

A person who has realised the Self or God, has broken the cycle of death and rebirth, and proceeds to live on one of the several spiritual planets in the spiritual sky. These planets are self-illuminated, that is, they have no sun and moon or days and nights, etc. One's life here is eternal, and full of knowledge and bliss. In this way, the person becomes one with God through identity, since God is described to be *Sat-Chit-Ananda* (eternal, full of knowledge, and full of bliss). Not going into further details on the subject here anymore, we shall turn to other methods which can bring liberation from falsehood and break the cycle of further incarnations.

The Method of Dreams

When we come to describe other methods, I find the method of dreams to be most important; it extends from the Vedic period to the present day scientific world, and it has been referred to by almost all methodologists in some form or the other.

In his analysis of the living being, Martinus found that there are three unshakable realities: (i) that which experiences life, that is "the I", (ii) the I's creative faculty, and (iii) the principle of "the created", that is its experiences or day-consciousness. These three principles are absolutely inseparable; if one of them did not exist, the other two would fall out immediately. This is the "triune principle" of Martinus which is analogous to the Vedic triplet "the seer, the seeing and the seen", as described by Sri Aurobindo too. "As none of these principles can be identical with a result of creation, the immortality of the living being becomes thereby evident as a fact... As these three principles constitute precisely the three conditions that must be fulfilled by a thing in order that it can appear 'living', every living being thus becomes identical with 'an eternally living thing'. This, in turn, means that the living being constitutes a reality that senses, experiences and manifests in an eternally continuing existence or experience of life." (Martinus 1933, 16-17) The terrestrial human being, however, has no conscious realisation of this eternal existence.

The faculty to remember in the terrestrial human being is almost completely at its latent stage in its cosmic cycle. When one does not remember events of this physical lifetime, it is simply a matter of course that one does not remember the events and details of the experiences one would have had further back in time. It is simply an evidence of an inadequate memory and it does not mean that one's past lives did not exist. There are centres in the brain which are connected through nerves to the physical sensory organs, such as seeing, hearing, smelling, etc. If this nerve is cut, the physical experiences will still be taking place but the person will not have a perception of the happenings. If this nerve is not cut, the perception of physical happenings will be as usual. In the same way, there are connections with "I" to the memories of the past lives; the memories being copies of the experiences which the individual would have had in previous lifetimes. Whenever these connections are revived, by one method or the other, the individual has an experience of bliss and one directly experiences the copies (memories) of the past happenings. One becomes conscious of the memories of one's previous existences. One's self-experienced realisation of immortality can at best be expressed as a beautiful vague impression, an instinct, a theory or a supposition. Such an experience is called a "spiritual experience", and the state in which it takes place is the one where "awake day-consciousness" of the individual borne by his physical body becomes borne by one of its other bodies. When such a transference takes place, the physical sensory perception of the individual is lost and he becomes unconscious on the physical plane. According to Martinus, this transference is identical to what we call "death".

The kind of transference described above can also take place in milder forms, such as anaesthetisation, fainting, hypnosis, trance or sleep. The day-consciousness is transferred from physical body to the "body of feeling", and since the person is still living, the day-consciousness can be brought back to the physical body. But, since the "body of memory" cannot transfer the experiences from "feeling" to "day-consciousness", the spiritual experiences thus perceived will, therefore, remain only in the unconscious state. However, at times, the transference of consciousness from day-consciousness to spiritual state is not perfect and consequently one finds oneself in an intermediate stage between the physical and spiritual. Examples of such "intermediate stages" are the situations under fever, disease, drugs, etc. Under such circumstances spiritual memories get merged with physical memories and enter into the day-consciousness of the person when one is physically awake. Such a fusion of the spiritual and physical memories is called a "dream". For a normal person, these dreams may be unreliable to a certain degree. "But to the developed cosmic being, who consciously, or by means of his will, can carry out these transformations of the day-consciousness from one body of manifestation to the other, and whose body of memory appears in a somewhat more pronounced constellation to the body of gravity and the body of feeling than that of the terrestrial human being, these spiritual experiences are not 'dreams' but fully awake experiences and thereby conscious facts." (Martinus 1933, 20)

The experience of "I" with life is determined by a general organ for each basic energy corresponding to the plane of existence (*see* Table 1). Six general organs (corresponding to six planes from the bottom) of I will be identical with one body for each plane of existence. On physical plane, physical body is most developed while other bodies are more or less latent; accordingly, I is most conscious to physical vibrations and least conscious to spiritual vibrations. The physical world is most real to him. Later in evolution, when the person reaches higher planes which are vibrating with spiritual energy, the situation is reversed. One becomes most conscious of the spiritual plane of existence and one's physical perception becomes latent. This transference of consciousness can be visualised in "dreams", the spiritual experiences can be stablised and one can trace one's origin back to spiritual worlds.

Hindu philosophy has always given importance to dreams as a means of attaining spiritual ends. According to Swami Sivananda Radha (1992, 148), a German psychiatrist having adopted a Hindu name during her discipleship in India, one is able to contact one's Higher Self, the Guru within, in dreams. Discipline coming with the understanding of one's own dreams brings independence from the criticism of others and from habitual self-assessment, there is awareness of new dimension. Swami Radha recommends the maintenance of a daily diary in which the dreams should be recorded immediately after awakening. He should keep a pen, paper and light ready for recording. Just before going to sleep, he should repeat at least twice to himself that he would remember the dream and write it down. The dream should be recorded whether he remembers it fully or partially, along with the events that took place and/or the mental preoccupation before the dream. He should pay attention to the changing perception of time and space by the mind during sleep. It is advisable to make one's own dictionary of symbols seen in dreams. Instead of consulting a book or following a particular school on symbols, it is better to know the way the mind expresses itself over and over again in symbols, which are very personal to the individual. It would be seen that dreams occur on different levels and gradually one begins to understand them clearly and directly.

In *Recovering Spirituality from Dreams,* Henry Reed (1995, 39) talks about his article "Getting Help From Dreams" and says, "It was about my initiation into the higher power of dreams by alcoholism. A turning point was a dream encounter with an old wise man who pointed to a bottle of wine and indicated that it was soul bait... The founders of Alcoholics credit Carl Jung for the gift of the secret formula, *spiritus contra spiritum,* Spirit against Spirits." According to Reed, every adversity has within itself a spiritual teacher ready to initiate the sufferer. He advises everyone to find some attachment (any will do) from which they could recover a spiritual gift.

In *Your Dream of Recovery: Dream Interpretation and the 12 steps,* which has much in common with the material presented in *Edgar Cayce and the 12 Stepping Stones to Spirituality,* Shelly Marshall says, "The purpose lurking behind events, or hovering over them, can often be revealed in dreams." (Reed 1995, 39) She has presented several examples in her book, including her personal stories. Her book begins with the following prayer, "God, grant me the serenity to accept all guidance revealed through my dreams, the courage to change the things I'm asked to, and the wisdom to interpret according to your will for me." According to Marshall, religion is only a bridge to spirituality; one should not worship the bridge, but cross it over and live in spirit. She draws a special connection between dreaming and drinking. She points out that our interpretation of dreams is ego-heroic and we wish to conquer the dream with our interpretation. The dream is discarded and interpretation is kept. One should learn the humility to respect a dream on its own merits and the focus should always be on finding God's will. She suggests methods to find something usable from a dream. Presence of puns has been mentioned in many dream books. According to Marshall, pun-consciousness in dreams can reveal many secrets, such as, "Alaska" is not the same as "I'll ask her", "sober" is not the same as "somber", "won" is not the same as "one", etc.

In *Your Dreams: God's Neglected Gift*, Herman Riffel (1981) has presented some useful pieces of information. According to him, in two or three seconds between the "tick" and alarm, a story was unravelled that took a long time to tell, and much longer to write. In comparison, an hour's dream must contain volumes of material. (p.10) He found that unending references to dreams (while asleep) and visions (while awake) were not only in the *Old Testament* but in the *New Testament* too. Abraham, Jacob, Joseph, Gideon and Solomon were led or encouraged by dreams. Joseph and Daniel could save their nations because they could interpret dreams correctly. Messages to prophets came through dreams and visions. For example, God said to Moses, "Hear now my words: If there is a prophet among you, I the Lord shall make Myself known to him in vision. I shall speak with him in a dream." (12:6) Major events of the *Bible* hinged on dreams and visions. He discovered that about one-third of the *Bible* is related to dreams and visions. (p.12) In his view, God still speaks to us in dreams and visions but the Western world has taken a negative and unbelieving attitude, though the Eastern world accepted dreams and visions many centuries ago.

According to Plato, there were three valid sources of knowledge: (i) five senses (seeing, hearing, smelling, touching and tasting), which is common with animals, (ii) reason, which is above animals, and (iii) spiritual realm, which he called "divine madness". However, Plato's successor Aristotle and his followers ruled out the validity of spiritual realm and "this humanistic philosophy was transmitted throughout the Western world". (Riffel 1981, 13) On his travels to the Eastern worlds, Riffel found that temple gods on every street corner and every important building were closely related to their religion, which indicated oneness between the spiritual and the physical worlds. To the Westerners, this seemed far-fetched and even ridiculous. Discoveries of Riffel shook the secure foundations of his Protestant Evangelical tradition.

Coming to dream interpretations by Riffel, he dreamt one day, "Alone in my car, I was following a bus down a dirt road, and the bus threw so much dust in the air, I could hardly see where I was driving." He had learned that a bus in dream represents the crowd and dust indicated confusion. His wife Lillie said, "The lord seems to be telling you to follow Him instead of the crowd." Riffel noted that as he opened himself to this new freshness, his inner spiritual life was quickened. According to him, God continued to press him harder. The turning point came and he had to decide whether he wanted to continue in the ministry of the church or open up to the mystery of healing independently. As he was unable to decide, a local artist in a group of people who sought the guidance of Holy Spirit, had this vision, "I see a beautiful belt that has many fingers proceeding out from it and hair like projections from the fingers." A woman received a word of knowledge that this vision concerned Lillie and Riffel, who were present in the group. They were not to be bound, even by a belt that was beautiful. They were to be free. Later, the artist told that the belt was a Protestant denomination, the fingers were the churches, and the hairlike projections from the fingers were people. In the words of Riffel, "God would let us be a blessing to many within the belt, but we were not to hold on to it. We were to let go in an attitude of humility." (pp.20-21) This is how Riffel got the evidence that God uses dreams and visions to speak to people. Eventually, he was dismissed as a pastor from the church. Although being fired from his job was a painful experience, both of them were now free and peaceful and were looking forward to the exciting new life God had promised.

God continued to guide Riffel and speak to him through dreams. One night, he had the following dream, "He was pushing a baby carriage with a little baby in it. When he came to the end of the street, he did not stop but pushed the carriage right up over a two-storey house. The house was like the one they were living in at the time. Once, he even lifted the carriage over his head, and the baby fell out, but he caught it." His friend, Francis Whiting explained that the dead end of the street represented the "dead end" of his ministry in the church. But he was not to stop, rather he was to carry the baby (new idea or concept) right up over the top of the traditional house in which his soul was then living. Even if the baby fell out, he would not lose it (the new idea). This was a very meaningful dream to him. He believed that the death and resurrection process spoken of by Jesus was being pointed out to him in his dreams, after he had opened himself to the Spirit.

Riffel found that his desire to know more about dreams was diminishing. Then, one night, he dreamt, that "he was on a raft some distance from the shore where people were swimming. The water was deep. A young girl who was in his care, fell off the raft and sank into the water. He dived, grabbed her and pulled her out of water". The dream interpreted meant that the baby (new idea) had now grown into a young girl and he was neglecting her (the truth). He became more alert and paid attention to it. He thought of the Jung Institute at Switzerland, got the scholarship in a miraculous way, and he and Lillie joined it to learn dream psychology. He was further guided in a dream wherein he entered a castle by crossing a moat around it. The moat meant the motherly containment. So, he broke the strong and perhaps dependent ties to his mother, freeing himself to be more masculine and aggressive. Earlier, when he asked God for a wife, a thought came to his mind to look at the school yearbook. He did so and stopped at the picture of Lillie. He proposed to her and soon they got married.

Sometimes, there are short dreams, but they can be very meaningful. A man in Switzerland came to him and told him about two little pictures he saw in dreams. In the first, he saw his left leg badly swollen and the veins running like dark lines. In the second, he saw a poisonous spider sitting on his briefcase. On being asked if there was anything wrong about his walking, his behaviour or his way of living, the man admitted that he had a messy situation in life, but he thought that it would remain under cover. Then, on being asked what he used the briefcase for, he said, "My profession." Riffel then told him that his bad behaviour may even affect his work. The man used to think that his behaviour was not bad, but after the dream interpretation he was shocked, and so he changed.

According to Riffel, if properly handled, the interpretation of dreams can bring a balance and wholeness in people. (p.60) He cites the example of King David of the *Old Testament*, who had the masculine and feminine qualities properly balanced. He was physically very strong and he defeated his son Absalom in a battle, when the latter wanted to oust the former from the throne. David wept bitterly for losing his loving son and was about to lose the battle, but for his wise general Joab. A study of the *Gospels* can reveal that Jesus had such a nice balance of authoritative strength and quiet gentleness. I have talked in greater length about the balance of male and female principles in a person as the prerequisite for Self-realisation. (Kumar 1997, 1998)

Riffel has given many more examples of his own dreams that guided him, along with examples of other people who later came to consult him. His work shows the importance of dreams and the way of interpretation, which can tell one the will of God and provide guidance and help from time to time. In his opinion, there are three reasons why we do not remember dreams: (i) we have been taught from the beginning that dreams are unimportant or irrelevant, (ii) we experience mechanical loss as we plunge into the affairs of the world on awakening, and (iii) spiritually, if one wants to keep God out of thoughts, His guidance goes unused. However, the dreams may continue in the form of nightmares. God may be trying to tell us something, if we care to listen and heed. The message is generally twofold; one, it may tell about the present situation of the dreamer, and two, what would happen if one continues in the present direction of affairs. The response received from dreams is proportional to the attitude shown towards them.

Carl Gustav Jung, perhaps the greatest exponent of dream analysis, said that dreams depict the inner state of the individual, and if properly analysed, they provide the real opportunity for growth. In *Man and His Symbols*, one can read his wonderful theory of anima and animus and the four stages of inner developments. (Jung 1964) Dreams should not be taken with their literary meaning, but they should be analysed to know oneself in the context of the outer circumstances. One cannot make a dictionary of symbols and their meanings as such, to be used by everyone. One should make one's own dictionary after writing them regularly and reviewing them at regular intervals. Nevertheless, a general guidance on symbols and their meanings can always be had from the writings of the experienced ones, as in the following.

Symbols and Their Meanings

Birds: Thoughts, ideas, spirituality – because birds fly in the sky, their appearance in dream shows the exalted mental conditions of the dreamer. The person is peaceful, pure and tranquil, especially if one dreams of a pigeon or a dove. One may be involved in philosophical or spiritual activities or in some creative venture.

Animals: Appearance of an animal shows a parallel mental/emotional state of the dreamer, according to the characteristics of the animal. For example, a rat which is known for entering the kitchen as a thief, may represent the entrance of the dreamer's thoughts at the lower levels of life. A cat may represent the destructions of ideas, a dog may represent faithfulness in his life, a fox may represent cunningness in the thoughts of the dreamer, a bull may represent hard-working nature of the person or presence of hard-work at the moment, according to the physical/mental/emotional condition during the period of dreaming. I once dreamt of running in a street, being chased by a dog, who finally caught up with me and bit me in the leg. Those were the days I was having some unpleasant arguments with my relatives on property matters, and sometimes there were embarrassing situations. The dream was a warning of such situation. Riffel once dreamt of catching a fish, which he could spear, but he said that he had no licence. In real life, his ministry was growing privately with some groups which were not officially sponsored by a church. The dream suggested that he had to use caution and not aggression in accepting invitations to go to churches without official authorisation. Thus, there is no fixed rule, one has to draw conclusions according to the circumstances in real life.

Snake: Appearance of a serpent in the dream denotes "sexual energy" according to one school of thoughts and "wisdom" according to another. I would say that both of them are correct when understood rightly. In Yoga tradition, repeated appearances of snake symbolise the "Spiritual Energy *Kundalini*" which corresponds to sex initially, and to wisdom after the conquest of sex by the individual.

House: Sometimes one is taken to the childhood house, representing the inner psychological house of good or bad memories, according to the mood of the dream. Often, we see a new house with many rooms, suggesting the development of newer levels of learning or consciousness, leading to gradual enlightenment. Old or broken house may suggest a gloomy situation in life. A good house may suggest a happy situation in life.

Automobiles: A new and big car may suggest an expression of freedom in one's life. If one is driving one's own car, it may mean that one is in control of one's own affairs. If someone else is driving it, it may be indicating the control of one's affairs by another person and a suggestion to achieve freedom for real progress and happiness.

Baby: New idea or thought.

People: Different persons in a dream do not have a literary meaning as such; they, in fact, represent parts of our own personality by their personal characteristics. If one sees a known person who is aggressive by nature, it may be suggesting that the dreamer is behaving aggressively these days in general, or perhaps to a particular person or to a situation in life. Dreaming of a peaceful person or a saint may be suggestive that the dreamer is internally turning peaceful or saintly. Seeing a police officer, a leader or any kind of authoritative person is suggestive that the dreamer has a part of his personality authoritatively taking charge of some affairs or situation of his life. Seeing a person as a saint or sitting in a meditative posture or as a *yogi* may indicate that that person has actually crossed across the spiritual boundaries. I personally know instances of this kind.

Beating/Killing: If one beats or kills a person in a dream, it may be suggestive that one is not happy with someone or with some situation in life and a settling of score is desired.

Loving: Loving someone in a dream normally means that the person has a loving attitude towards others.

Sex: A widely misunderstood dream. It does not mean that the dreamer is having sexual relations with someone. It certainly means that the dreamer is having an interaction with one's inner self or creative part and is approaching a balance between the masculine and feminine principles, that is intellectuality and sentimentality. When properly understood, it brings a feeling of joy and fulfilment, rather than guilt. However, homosexual and lesbian relations in a dream (as well as in real life) show an imbalanced and unnatural part of the person. The individual may be looking for his lost part of the personality and thus achieve a balance. But unnatural relations cannot make up for the loss, one has to find the lost part by learning and healing.

Money: Getting money, a purse or a treasure in a dream is indicative of energy or power in real life, because of its buying capacity. Loss, on the other hand, is indicative of a weaker situation in real life.

Clothes: The type of clothing worn in a dream is indicative of wearing such a dress in real life, suggestive of how one likes to appear before others.

Naked: Seeing oneself without any clothes in a dream indicates that one is exposed to others and there may be some embarrassment. It may also mean that one is hiding nothing from God or from those before whom one is exposed.

Triangle, square, circle or ball: It is indicative of the inner wholeness in the dreamer.

Water: An important symbol that appears in different forms, such as a pool, a river, an ocean and so on. Clean water indicates good consciousness in real life, leading to philosophical or religious perfection. Muddy or unclear water may suggest a messy or nuclear situation in real life; one may be looking for a way out in some confused situation of life. Crossing a river is a sign of no return, which one has crossed from the physical to the spiritual dimension. Such a person is supposed to have graduated from the school of earth.

A female figure appearing in the dreams of males is called "anima" and the male figure appearing in the dreams of females is called "animus" by Carl Jung. (1964, 158-159) The purpose of anima or animus is to guide and bring perfection in the individual towards wholeness. The figure also improves with the improvement of the person. Although a detailed discussion has already been given earlier (Kumar 1997, 1998), the four levels are briefly reproduced here:

Anima

Level 1 : Primitive woman, symbolising ignorance, for example, Eve.

Level 2 : Romanticised beauty, such as Cleopatra, Helen of Troy, etc., symbolising sex.

Level 3 : Virgin Mary, breast feeding the child Christ, symbolising love.

Level 4 : The Greek goddess of wisdom – Athena, Mona Lisa – wearing a mysterious smile, Sapienta, or Shulamite in the song of Solomon, Devi Durga or *Shakti*, all pointing towards spiritual experience.

Animus

Level 1 : The wholly physical man, the fictional jungle man Tarzan.

Level 2 : The "romantic man", ranging from the 19th century British poet Shelley or the "man of action" to America's Ernest Hemingway, war hero, hunter, etc.

Level 3 : The bearer of the "word" – Lloyd George, the great political orator.

Level 4 : The wise guide to spiritual Truth – often projected on to Mahatma Gandhi, Jesus Christ or Buddha.

The fourth stage is rarely achieved by the people in modern times, but it is not too difficult for serious students of Truth. I also witnessed their appearance in that order as detailed earlier. (Kumar 1998)

Eckankar is called the "Religion of Light of Sound" and it is based on dreams and soul travel experiences. With its headquarters in Minneapolis, Minnesota, the present leader, Sri Herald Klemp, induces dreams into his disciples and takes them to various planes of higher reality in dreams. There are a series of lectures called "dream discourses one" and "dream discourses two", through which monthly training and practice is provided to its students. There are several books in which experiences of travel to the remote pasts, such as the Mayan and Atlantis civilisations, are given.

My personal experiences with dreams: Although I have been seeing dreams all my life, I would mention here just a few in the recent years which provided life-changing spiritual guidance.

Sometime around the year 1980, I dreamt of flying high in the sky till I reached the summit of a hill, surrounded by beautiful lakes, meadows and gardens. Reaching the top of the hill, I saw a beautiful temple, absolutely white in colour and shining with equal luminosity from every side. It gave me an instant feeling of happiness and bliss and a longing to have further visits to such a place. This further increased my love towards God and led me to regular practice of yoga and meditation. It was the beginning of the withdrawal of my interests from the affairs of the world. Now I know that it was a temple on one of the astral planes.

Since then, I had regular dreams of the similar nature; flying over places similar to those on earth but without the negative attributes of earth. Lakes, mountains, rivers, gardens, fruits and flowers so lovely and soothing that you cannot describe the derivative happiness. I could fly over streets, colonies and houses; stop and descend on the ground if and when I liked, and take a fly-off again.

Once I saw myself standing in front of a translucent fortress having two gates and a water canal in the middle. People entered through one gate and came out of the other. People appeared to be circles of light, not in the form of physical bodies. There were people moving on the bank of the canal and also on the grass; they were however in the form of a point of light or a circle of light. I could see three persons on the ground; one of them instructed telepathically to move forward. Soon, I found myself crossing a very broad river like an ocean of clear blue water. I had no dimensions of my body, just a point of awareness. Having crossed the river, I found myself in front of a group of mountains. I was trying to look at one of the mountains when suddenly the dream came to an end. Perhaps it was an out-of-body travel by soul and I returned to the physical body on earth. It gave me a first-hand experience of the higher spiritual realms under the guidance of an invisible helper or a Guru. It could be the Eckankar Master, Sri Herald Klemp or Pythagoras or... Next day, I was full of happiness and my faith in yoga and meditation was further increased. This was in the year 1987.

I had several visits to such realms which were the source of happiness and bliss on one hand, and detachment from the world and its relations on the other.

Several dreams of snakes around me in different forms, without any feeling of fear, was almost a daily feature while I was asleep. In later days, I used to see snakes with open hoods in different situations. Sometimes, a snake would be looking at me in a friendly way, at another time it would be crawling on my body, yet at another time it would be flying with me in the sky. These were the dreams indicative of the awakening of *kundalini.*

In 1995, while I was in San Francisco, I dreamt of a big gathering in which I could see a person with an outstanding physique and a glow on the face and eyes, looking at me in a very affectionate way. He was moving in one direction and I read the name "Bapu" written on his chest. The next day, I came to know from my mother that it was the nickname of the present-day saint of India, Asaramji. As I understand now, it was my High Self coming to initiate and bless me in the form of a Guru.

Near-Death Experience

The term NDE and related experiences have been mentioned earlier. Two main contributors in this study are Dr. Raymond Moody and Professor Kenneth Ring. One gets a first-hand proof of the life beyond in an NDE through any one of the various situations, such as a surgical operation, falling from a mountain, a road accident, etc. My opinion is that getting the taste of after-life is like visiting a foreign country on a visitor's visa – which should be converted into the permanent residence or citizenship through meditative, metaphysical or any other method of Self-realisation. Such an experience is not related to any religion or only to good people. Most people, after an NDE, become more spiritual or begin to believe in some form of God. They lose fear of death, and in some cases, their intuitive or psychic abilities are found to be enhanced.

According to Atwater (1988), some people find it difficult to adjust to a normal life because of the profundity of the experience. Negative reactions include anger and disappointment due to return to life, fear and inability to talk about their experience, and depression in resuming their lives. Positive reactions include ecstasy and thrill of the wonderful experience, gratitude and awe for the happening, authority and humility with respect to fearlessness of death. "Ring, philosopher Michael Grosso, and others have theorised that the NDE may be a form of enlightenment or a 'gateway to a higher consciousness', and could have a transformative effect on the entire planet if enough people have similar experiences." (Guiley 1991, 400) Carol Zaleski (1987) opines that NDE stories can introduce a "religious sense of the cosmos" into the scientific or secular understanding of the individuals.

An important thing to be mentioned about an NDE is that it takes place by itself, if and when it happens, there is no specific method to induce it. Yet, however, there are factors in the psychological makeup in a person, such as abuse, neglect, dissociation in childhood, etc., which make a person prone to an NDE. Barbara Harris Whitfield is such an example. In her own words (Whitfield 1995, 25-28), "Then I separated from my body, just as I had when I was being abused as a child... I saw myself in a bubble, face down in my crib, crying just as hysterically... energy was wrapping around me and going through me, holding up every molecule of my being. It took me a long time to use the word God... in a cloud of bubbles... each bubble was another event from my life... I relived 32 years of my life... I could hear myself saying, 'No wonder, no wonder. No wonder you are the way you are now. Look what was done to you when you were a little girl.' I saw all the abuse... my mother physically abusing me came from the abuse that she had received as a child." While out-of-body during her NDE, Barbara heard two nurses talking about her and noticed that they did not change the pillows she did wet. After coming back in her body, she told the nurses all about their conversation and the fact that they did not change the wet pillows, which surprised the nurses. This description, and several others of this kind, should disprove the sceptics who believe that an NDE is a dream.

Barabara defines "spiritual awakening" as an experiential opening to a power greater than ourselves. (Whitfield 1995, XI) Martinus defined "spiritual knowledge" as an analysis of experiences that are promoted by forces that cannot be sensed by the ordinary physical senses. (Martinus 1933, 6) Both are authors who achieved Self-realisation at different times and through entirely different methods, yet, their conclusion is the same, and it is parallel to Eastern findings; see, for example, the work of Sri Aurobindo. Barabara became introduced to this spiritual energy "that can be called many things – *kundalini*, Divine Energy, Holy Spirit, *Ruach Ha Kodesh* (The Holy Wind) – that guides my life. When it is invited into your life, it will show you too how to see from a higher point of view". (Whitfield 1995, 15-16) In her view, a Mystic is someone who relates to God in direct experiential communion, through the soul or child within. One receives direct knowledge of reality, and most of our journeys lead to this reality. What a confirmation of the ancient Eastern beliefs and the findings of many seekers!

Diane Goble was awakened to the Reality of the Spiritual World after she slipped under the raging river and breathed in the cold water (from the cover page of her book *Through the Tunnel*). She believed that she was going to die and soon she was watching the scene of her death from above. Suddenly, she found herself speeding through a dark tunnel towards light. A Being of Light communicated with her telepathically and made her pass through a library of books through which she accumulated knowledge. Being given an option to stay back or return to earth to complete her mission, she decided to come back, though reluctantly, and dragged her body to the raft in the hydraulic waterfall, where she had sunk and had virtually died. This is a model story of an NDEer. The message she gave is, "We are all on our Spiritual Paths back to our Source. Earth life is an education and a creative opportunity – its purpose is to enhance our spiritual growth as Children of a Loving God." (Globe 1993, back cover) And again, "The pursuit of knowledge and wisdom should occupy our time – learning how to be *in* the physical world without becoming attached to its pleasures or caught up in its troubles. No matter what, it is only temporary." (Globe

1993, 36) Is it not exactly what Gautam Buddha said 2600 years ago, confirmed by his contemporaries, such as Zoroaster, Confucius, Pythagoras, etc., and then found independently and said by Jesus Christ? We discover the same "truth" over and over again, by different methods at different times.

An important observation by Diane Globe is, "The Clear Light is that which appears to everyone just prior to the moment of death, but few even see it." (Globe 1993, 33) According to her, love, kindness and compassion raise the frequency of the person. One can tolerate being as close to the Light as one has been open to the Light during one's physical lifetime. Complete liberation from negative *Karma* can be achieved by recognising the *Clear Light* and merging with it, but if one dies with hatred in the heart, one may not even see the Light. One will not reach its frequency and will go on to experience the Bardo. "Bardo Thodol" of Tibet says that the chance of illumination is greatest at the moment of death. According to the findings of Nils Bjorn Kvastad, in his *Problems of Mysticism,* "The deceased sees a lightning, called the 'clear light of the void'. If he unites with it and consciously realises it, he will have a mystical experience and be liberated." (Kvastad 1980, 351) In view of Kvastad, Dr. Raymond Moody may be talking of the same light of Bardo Thodol in his writings. "Mystical experience can then be a foretaste of life after death, a view the mystic and devotee of Isis, Apulejus, expressed when he said about a mystical experience: 'I have passed through the gates of death'. However, if this light is realised and the after-life has become a continuous mystical experience, as the 'Bardo Thodol' holds it can be, this is no individual, separate existence. The deceased will somehow be merged in the universe." (Kvastad 1980, 352) A *yogi*, at his experience of death while still living, sees this Light at a point, as it has been mentioned in my own experiences, and then, there is a series of visits to higher realms. (Kumar 1998)

Through Crisis and Suffering

Barbara has noted that (i) the Chinese symbol for crisis means opportunity, and (ii) ancient Eastern spiritual literature has always recognised that liberation can be achieved during crisis and suffering. (Whitfield 1995, 9) I would agree with this and add that whenever an individual advances spiritually, his physical conditions become more difficult, so much so that it appears like a sort of crisis. Paul Twitchell and Harold Klemp have given similar statements in their books on Eckankar. Once, the famous saint, Surdas, was offered a comfortable living with a house and servants by a rich devotee. He accepted it and the very first night, Lord Krishna appeared to him in a dream and said, "So your spiritual quest has come to an end?" Surdas was alarmed; he immediately left the house and continued moving from place to place, singing devotional songs to Lord Krishna as before, and imparting knowledge to the world. Hence, the condition of crisis seems to be a pre-requisite for spiritual development, whether it comes by itself or is created through efforts. I can further confirm this through my personal experiences. Once liberation or Self-realisation has been achieved, it does not matter how one lives.

Childbirth is an opportunity for women during which some of them are known to leave their bodies and view the delivery from a high point in the room. Some of them have reported the presence of deceased relatives, some have visited the landscapes on higher realms and some of them experienced unbelievable ecstasy which is followed by bliss for many days or even weeks. These are spiritual experiences which should be allowed to happen through awareness and relaxation if the women are prepared for it in advance. Christian Graff, founder of the Kundalini Research Network in California, is a brilliant example in this context; she got her awakening at the birth of her second child. Later, she took a formal initiation from Swami Muktananda in Honolulu.

Bereavement is a crisis in which someone, who is excessively attached to a person on the deathbed, can experience awakening. I know some people personally, to whom this has happened. I can also cite the example of my father who expired on 7 September, 1992. I was at the university in Fiji at that time and I arrived in Delhi on 13 September. On 7 September, it was around 8 in the evening that I was doing my regular prayer and meditation in Fiji. I got an exceptional concentration and experienced peace for about an hour and I felt the presence of someone around me during the whole hour. My father loved me more than I loved him and he never wanted me to leave India those days.

On 13 September, I wept bitterly in the room of my father on my arrival in Delhi. We slept late that night. In the early hours of the morning, I felt my shoulder shaken strongly by someone and I woke up. I felt a breathing around me and I knew that it was my father. I then said many things to him for about half-an-hour and assured him that I will take care of my mother and will see that the property left by him would be equally divided between all. I then requested him to wake me up once again later, to give me the proof of his presence. And he did wake me up once again that morning. The same night, my sister heard my father calling her name and she saw him standing outside the window for a few seconds in the suit I had brought for him from London. He was then thirty-five years old and was smiling.

The main point to tell here is that my mother was highly involved in the process of my father's death and she got the awakening in that period. Three days before his death, my father used to report the presence of some deceased relatives and friends standing around him. He also reported the presence of someone in a uniform, writing something in a notebook. He commented that this police man could not harm him in any way, since he had not committed any crime. He also reported seeing me wearing a white turban and involved in some ritual. This was the foreseeing of the event which took place a few days later. My mother was crying day and night and continued to do so until a few weeks later. Eventually, I brought my mother with me to Fiji where she stayed for a few months.

As we all noted, my mother would go into periods of trance now and then and would report seeing some deceased people around. She would see some strange writings on the wall which she could partially understand. Her meditation with chanting of *mantras* increased very much. She used to see celestial beings in the room specially when we were engaged in devotional songs and when I used to read or talk about a religious book. She used to offer food to Lord Krishna and she invariably reported His coming there in an astral body and sharing the food for a few seconds. She was a completely changed person now.

Sharing the dying moments of his wife Sally, the English mystic poet, P. J. Kavanagh, experienced "revelation" in the hospital in Java. In his own words, "It was not a visual experience, but it is best described in visual terms. It was as though streams of connections of light were going from cloud to cloud. Everything seemed connected. It was not an aural experience either, but if you can imagine choirs of angels, the music of the spheres, they were present. And what was really surprising about it was that there seemed enormous vats of consolation. Everything was all right, absolutely everything was all right. It was of immense warmth. This came as no surprise; it seemed as though one had always known that. And it was only afterwards that I realised that I hadn't thought, 'My goodness! This is a revelation, an illumination!'" (Lello 1985, 48) After about two months, he started seeing colours in a very heightened form, in a mysteriously vibrating way. He would suddenly feel overwhelming love for England, which he had never felt before.

Kavanagh was in his early sixties at that time. While attending a party, he was suddenly filled with a bubbling well of laughter; though not loud, it was an inexhaustible Mozartian kind of laughter. It was just a laughter, not at anyone, and there was no self in it. It was beautiful, and it subsided with an inner cleansing, just as one feels after a burst of weeping. It was a sudden release from the self. According to Kavanagh, it was the heightened emotional state which was responsible for the dropping of the barrier. He thinks that every man and woman has his/her own moment. For him, these were the moments of literary inspiration containing light and warmth; one feels human rather than personal. He does not think that these illuminations can be harnessed. However, some kind of formal concentration or social concentration, some form of prosaic habit is necessary. It led him to God in a new way. In his opinion, everybody has to find their own path.

Brutal Torture can make one feel the presence of God and induce transcendental knowledge from within. This is what happened to Dr. Sheila Cassidy of England in 1975 when she was arrested and brutally tortured by the Chilean secret police. On being asked about the moment when her belief became more profound, she replied that there wasn't a particular moment. She never had any experience of God speaking in words. It was more a knowledge from within. When they started to take off her clothes, she was completely incredulous because she had always thought that she had a measure of protection. But while it was happening, she did have some kind of sense of the presence of God which never left her. In her own words, "At the time of interrogation and the fear of rape, I was just surviving minute by minute and being absolutely terrified and not feeling any emotion for the people... after the torture, I was more and more convinced of a loving God who knew and loved me personally." (Lello 1985, 18-19)

Road to Damascus: According to Sir Fred Hoyle, F.R.S., scientist and astronomer, blinding revelation for scientists as well as for religious people comes through a "crisis". In his own words, "If we go back to the road to Damascus, St. Paul had been putting conditionals on his thinking and suddenly they were removed. This is why it is an intensely personal experience. It can only happen if one has gone through a sort of crisis either of moral, mathematical or scientific thinking." (Lello 1985, 32-33) In his opinion, everybody has to travel on the road to Damascus. Hoyle says that Einstein summed up the whole scientific philosophy in his remark, "God may be subtle but he's not malicious"; it is just a feeling within oneself, it's a light on the road to Damascus. As pointed out earlier, Sir Alister Hardy, F.R.S., commenting on the term "road to Damascus" used by Sir Fred Hoyle frequently in *Revelation – Glimpses of Reality,* said that the term means a "sudden revelation", or something very important, which influences the whole outlook of the individual and to which he might give the name of God. (Lello 1985, Preface)

Identification with Nature brought revelation to and changed the life of Jiddu Krishnamurti of India, who was groomed as imminent 'Word Teacher' by theosophists Annie Besant and C. W. Leadbeater in England. In his own words, "There was a man mending the road; that man was myself; the pickaxe he held was myself... I could feel the wind passing through the tree, and the little ant on the blade of grass, I could feel... I was in everything or rather everything was in me, inanimate and animate, the mountain, the worm and all breathing things." The next day, he experienced the following, "Such a profound calmness both in the air and within myself, the calmness of the bottom of a deep unfathombale lake. Like the lake, I felt my physical body with its mind and motions could be ruffled on the surface but nothing, nay nothing, could disturb the calmness of my soul... Nothing could ever be the same. I have drunk of the clear and pure waters at the source of the fountain of life and my thirst was appeased." (*Krishnamurti: The Years of Awakening* by Mary Lutyens, also Lello 1985, 57-58)

Krishnamurti did not believe in organised religions or a hierarchical attitude towards life. He rejected faith as a concept. In his opinion, one should begin with self-knowledge. The ancient Hindus, long before the Greeks, said, "Know Thyself." In knowing yourself, you are going beyond yourself. According to him, a Hindu, a Muslim or a Christian is a human brain which has been programmed like a computer. The 'truth' is interpreted by each one according to one's conditioning. Each one must be a light to one because freedom is necessary. The whole world is afraid of death. But the present or 'Now' contains all time. When one understands time and death in this way, one is living with death all the time and there is no fear of it. Krishnamurti said that 'truth' can't be put into words, just as the universe can't be put into a telescope. The immeasurable cannot be measured by words. In order to transcend the measurement one should meditate. In meditation, there is no comparison and one gets freedom from measurement.

Loneliness and Agony of Masturbation before males triggered the spiritual experience in British actress Sarah Miles. According to her, a male director can't tell a woman how to masturbate; something that we all do in private. Shortly after doing the scene of masturbation, she had her first revelation. On seeing the rushes, everybody said, "Well done," but Sarah was distressed because of the pain of the loneliness of doing it. Walking on the lonely road back home, she experienced, "It was quite beautiful. I had enormous heat coming from an area just above the solar plexus. It was a fierce heat from the center, like fire, hot fire, hotter even than fire. I also noticed that I was numb in my extremities, my feet were cold and I was icy but boiling in the centre. My breath seemed to be coming from a place that I had never known it came from before. I felt fear because of this heat and then it changed. I was doubtless. There was no doubt, there was an aching of strength that passeth all understanding. I felt at that moment, not I, but something else that was me, yet was not me, was capable of just dancing across estuary. I felt that I could, through something else that was happening to me, do anything. It was a moment of utter doubtlessness and I think almost omnipotence. It was as if God was within and without and I was at one within and without with all things. It sounds terribly clichéd, but it is so difficult to describe. Extraordinary doubtlessness. This was what was so strange – doubtlessness about everything and knowledge about everything." (Lello 1985, 75)

Sarah hears an inner voice all the time since then and she follows it. She realised that we are all eternal and she decided to discover her spiritual body and eternity. As she looks back, the actual moment of revelation was perhaps a split second, while the actual journey was about five minutes. Doubtlessness, Godliness and strange breathing remained after the experience. She passed from being all powerful to being a total puppet. Something else took over her which was telling her things to do. After reaching home, she was in a hot bath for almost three days, constantly topping it up with hot water. She was being drawn towards death and she had no fear of it in her. Something happened to her and she took a handful of sleeping pills to swallow, then a realisation came and she put the pills aside, she took a pen and paper and wrote away, wrote away for three years, as she says. It led her to meditation and yoga, both of which have served her beautifully over the years. In her opinion, meditation is a wonderful route for people in order to gain self-knowledge. Sarah put herself in the hands of fate, which she had never done before. She knew that death was not the end. It was not a belief – it was knowledge, she knew it. But she feels that putting this knowledge into practice is an extremely hard work. Sarah received a large amount of correspondence in response to her revelation programme. She was happy that her programme was helpful in awakening the seeds of spirituality which have lain dormant in most people.

Hurtling Downhill, being catapulted down head over heels, heading towards a big drop, Britain's best known mountaineer Doug Scot thought, "Well I am now going to die but it won't be a bad thing! A warm feeling came over me. Then I stopped dead in the snow." (Lello 1985, 94) He experienced what it is like being in an avalanche, having visions of snow and rocks, and the episode left something permanent in him. He realised that, although he would not like to die now, he was not afraid to die. A few weeks later, Doug was walking with a woman who was suffering enormous grief by the death of her boyfriend, mountaineer Dougal. Suddenly, he felt vibrations in the landscape and a rush of energy on the periphery of his vision. The intensity of experience gave a lot more compassion to him than he had even before. He could understand people's problems and could see a connection between everything. He had a very heightened perception which was hard to describe. Although it lasted for a few seconds only, it changed the whole outlook of his life. He would get involved with friends and acquaintances having problems and was effective in helping them with support, sympathy, understanding and awareness; earlier, he was ineffective. For the first time, he started doing something for someone else without expecting any reward.

The experience lifted him up to a new way of looking at the whole business of being alive. He got interested in the literature on the topic and he calmed himself down because of its profundity. He started reading all kinds of esoteric literature, Tao, I Ching and a lot more in search of knowing what it was. Although the effect was strong for a few months only, it remained a reference point for him for all time to come. Although nothing happened to him on the mountain, Doug noted that one did not eat or sleep much there and that might be a key to the heightened sensory perception. One could feel the thoughts coming, and there was a space between the thoughts. That space contained calm and peace. Although he was not in that space all the time, he valued the experience as a permanent reference point. However, he maintains that one did not have to go to mountains to have such an experience, one could have it at the back of one's garden if one knew the technique and if one had the burning desire. I would agree with Doug on this, since one can have the same experiences through meditation sitting in one's own house.

On being asked if he hoped to have one of those moments of revelation again, he said that it would be great if it happened, but one does not get it when one tries too hard for something. It is only when one lets go of the ambition to climb a peak that events often work to allow one to get there. How true it is, as I can say so with my own experiences! It is the perfecting of the means and not the result, that the result is seen coming out. Doug Scott could control his body to an extent that he could heal himself. He could sense the needs of others on meeting them by becoming calm, relaxed, interested and sympathetic to them. He has realised the truth in the saying of Ouspensky that 'most of us are asleep' and in the saying of Gurdjieff that 'most of us live in the state of sleep'. Doug is shocked on awakening to his own faults and on getting the glimpse of the vast potential which each one of us has.

A finding similar to that of Doug Scott is written by Harold Klemp of Eckankar in his letters of Light and Sound. A woman parachuter could not see her parachute opening up, in spite of her best efforts. Seeing imminent death, she happened to come out of her body and then she found that she had forgotten to press a particular button. Immediately, she entered her body, pressed the required button and safe-landed later. The heightened perception she had while she was out of her body changed her whole view of life, and she was not the same person again. She eventually took to metaphysics and serious meditation, and reported improving spiritually as time passed.

Knocked Down Completely by a Warrant Officer at the Japanese Prisoner of War Camp, Sir Laurens Van Der Post suddenly heard a voice inside him which said, "Go back and let him beat you again!" (Lello 1985, 118) He turned instantly and stood before the officer. The officer picked up the chair on which he was sitting and just when he was about to hit, a thought came in his mind that he had just knocked this man down. The rhythm of something evil in him was broken down, he threw the chair away and walked away in disgust. Post is certain that if he had not done this, a lot of people would have been killed that day, but he had no knowledge that he was going to do it. In his opinion, the voice saying 'go back' was the voice of creation. He has always felt that there is something in us, whether we die or not, which is always just a jump ahead of death. And it was the voice of creation, he felt, speaking at that moment. Born in South Africa, he has written more than twenty books and has made several films including *The Story of Carl Gustav Jung*.

Sir Laurens observes that the scientists forget the quote of Einstein that 'the spirit of science is devout' and they fail their own calling. Science tends to reduce the spirit to rationalism, which, in his opinion, is wrong. He thinks that this overall drive is in everyone and we can make ourselves receptive to revelation. There is something in life which tries to compensate, if life goes too far in one direction. The Spirit speaks to different people in different ways. One cannot explain the artist, priest or a scientist rationally. We cannot rationally find out the element behind their creativity; for example, something that made Archimedes discover that the amount of water displaced by his body in a bath is equal to the mass of the body. Descartes said, 'I think, therefore I am,' which means that there is "something" which thinks through us. The Germans call it *einfall* – an inspiration – that falls into us suddenly like a flash of light, and an unknown thought is suddenly recognised. According to Sir Laurens, revelation is a flashing act of recognition. However, he thinks that revelation is continuous, it need not be dramatic always. He has more faith in evolutionary revelation than the startling and dramatic ones. He observes that man has never felt so threatened, insecure and frightened as at present because of the terrible fear of the atom bomb. It is the force created by us, but we do not know how to control it. It is this imbalance which has produced insecurity.

Insult Turned Loving Embrace evoked the revelation of the old proverb, *"Forgive us our trespasses, as we forgive them that trespass against us,"* in the heart of British actor and comedian Kenneth Williams who was serving the military in Sri Lanka. Having thrown out the Indians from the British mess, he was asked later by his officer to go in their mess in proper uniform and apologise to the Indian officer for his act. While doing so, he was feeling very ashamed and degraded and expected insult in return. But the Indian officer embraced him, kissed him on both cheeks and invited him to have food with them. Later, when Kenneth expressed surprise, the Indian officer reminded him of their own old proverb. In his own words, "I was thunderstruck and transfixed. It was a revelation for me because I'd said it a hundred times without any real concept of the import of the words." (Lello 1985, 128) It came as a bolt from the blue, he became aware of the real significance of the Lord's Prayer by a foreigner. Then he came to understand the meaning of "goodbye", which was "God be with you". He re-examined and realised how important it was.

According to Kenneth, self-will has a purpose which science cannot explain. Science can give the "how" of electricity being harnessed or occurring of lightening, but it cannot explain "why". Faith supplies the answer to "why". In his opinion, comedy has a mystical content. A mysterious thing happens in an auditorium where laughter is created. One can convert a misery-making thing into an amusing and creative thing through comedy. In his view, happiness is an ephemeral thing and the most we can hope to achieve is a contenment with our lot.

Revelations was a television series in Britain in the early 80's, which produced a large correspondence showing that the writers experienced something beyond the ordinary and yet quite real. The varieties included sudden appreciation of beauty or love, a new understanding of events and an immediate knowledge of appropriate action. Alister Hardy Research Center at Oxford examined more than four thousand experiences and published the report. They speak of "significant links between direct religious experience and such factors as personal happiness, meaningfulness of life, lack of materialism and high levels of social responsibility. They suggest that most people associate the experience with a spiritual awareness. In whatever way revelation is experienced, it seems to be largely ignored by church and science." (Lello 1985, 135) The saddest observation was that the people could not talk about their experiences to anyone. Those who were supposed to provide the guidance were not able to help, understand or explain. Those who have not had similar experiences would always disregard them in one way or the other; nevertheless, the experiencers were certain of the truth seen and that they have a greater world within them than what the ordinary senses can perceive. Thus, a spiritual experience appears to be personal and beyond ordinary senses. According to Lello, the experience is like a signpost or beacon which points the way and indicates the existence of a spiritual domain which can be trusted.

Through Sexual Energy

It is the most powerful, most natural and perhaps the *shortest path* to Self/God-realisation, if it is understood properly. "The *Tantriks* tried to transform sex into spirituality, but the preachers of morality in our country did not allow the message to reach the masses." (Rajneesh, n.d. 151) Although thinking about *tantra* was banned thousands of years ago, its philosophy is immortalised in the monuments of Khajuraho and the temples of Puri and Konark. On seeing the images of naked couples in intercourse on the outer walls of the temples of Khajuraho in India, one does not feel any sense of vulgarity, rather, one is enveloped in the feelings of sacredness and peace. On the faces of the statues, one will find the serene and peaceful impression of Buddha and Mahavira. The statues were created by the visionaries who knew spiritual sex intimately. Even as watching two men fight satisfies and dissipates the instinct of fight deep-rooted in a man, meditation on these images of intercourse evaporates mad sexuality from inside the watcher and he becomes calm and peaceful. Freedom from lust can be achieved through long sessions of concentration on these drawings. On freeing oneself from the sexuality of the outer walls and on entering the temple, one sees the peaceful statue of Lord Shiva instituted inside. This is the secret of *tantra.*

Talking about *samadhi*, Lord Jesus said, "There shall be time no longer." If one observes the process of copulation and orgasm closely, one would find that two things are created in those depths – egolessness and timelessness; and these are the characteristics of *samadhi.* In that brief moment of sexual climax, the individual tastes bliss and divinity. To have the same experience again, the person indulges in sex repeatedly and loses a considerable amount of energy and vitality. One later regrets one's indulgence and laments the loss. However, one has touched the subtler level of the sexual experience which is *religious* in essence. What one has to understand, at this point, is that "sexual pleasure" is not the "end" but the "means" to attain the permanent bliss of *samadhi.* Normally, ejaculation accompanies orgasm. If one can know the secret of separating "ejaculation" from "orgasm", one will not lose the energy and vitality on one hand, and enjoy the "bliss" of the Absolute on the other. This is what happens to the yogis. They are in a state of permanent bliss and full of energy. This is where *meditation* comes into the picture and one is required to know the art of converting sex into meditation.

Muhammad Subuh, later known as Pak Subuh and nicknamed Bapak, was a Muslim Sufi, a native of Java. According to him, interaction on the human level comes about through sexual intercourse. He believed that the "act of sexual union gives man a chance to be influenced by the force which is properly human because, in the moment of orgasm, the innermost self of the man or woman become isolated from the lower forces. At this instant, if a man can be free of desire, and of thinking, he will become aware of an inner awakening to his true nature". (Bacrot 1976, 108) When one's consciousness is raised to a purely human level in the sexual act, one can become aware of the nature of the lower forces and can detach oneself from them. Once their domination is over, the person becomes their master and then he can direct them into their proper paths.

According to Swami Satyananda Saraswati (1984), "spiritual energy" passes through four different levels of existence: ignorance, sex, love and spiritual experience. In the process of yoga, when *kundalini* reaches the fourth centre at the level of heart, energy is converted from sex to love, and when *kundalini* reaches the sixth centre between the eyebrows, the energy is converted from love to spiritual experience. Thus, in yoga, one's endeavour is to transform sexual energy into love and then to spiritual experience. Pundit Gopi Krishna (1975) opined that it is the same energy which is at the two extremes of existence: at the lower level, it is responsible for the erotic experience, while at the higher level it gives rise to spiritual experience. The two levels are so close to each other that they appear barely separable form one another.

Elisabeth Haich talks, in depth, about "sexual energy" and shows the way to convert it into the highest consciousness through yoga. "Sexuality and the highest consciousness are two different forms in which the one divine creative force, the Logos, is manifested. Sexual energy, the lowest form of the Logos, can in man become the highest form of Logos, divine consciousness... Modern depth psychology can help us along a part of this path of development, but only yoga and meditation can bring us to the goal." (Haich 1982, 17-18) Freud too observed that sexuality can be converted into "spiritually creative power" and he called the process *sublimation.* Haich points out that the only fuel which is absolutely indispensable for the stimulation of the *chakras* is "sexual energy". The whole process is equally valid for both sexes. The same sexual energy, which has brought man from spiritual state to body, can bring him back to his divine primal state of wholeness. It is loneliness and not personal relations which pave the way to God. Yoga is the healthiest and shortest path to God. One cannot give up sex unless one has known fully what a healthy sex life means. The secret key to the philosopher's stone of the alchemists is one's own sexual energy.

According to Elisabeth, an individual is nothing but one's own sexual energy, which passes through various stages and assumes different forms. "As long as man remains unconscious, he experiences God within himself as sexual desire. When he has become conscious, he experiences God as his own *Self*, as his now true being, as *I am*! God is, for man, the absolute *state of self-awareness.*" (Haich 1982, 49) She terms the union of *Logos* and consciousness of the physical being as *mystical marriage.* Her book shows a picture representing God in Ancient Mexico: at the base is a serpent, symbolising sexual energy; on it stands a man's figure which symbolises the body sustaining, emotional, mental and intuitive manifestations; at the very top is the incorporeal, pure spiritual and radiant self-awareness: God. She has noted that the same serpent in India is known as *kundalini,* and has described the manifestation of the energy at the seven levels called *chakras.*

It is sexual energy alone which brings us liberation from itself and frees us from the very sexual desires. It is the cause of inner unrest and it continually goads us to find the inner path. "In an unexpected moment, among the animal impulses, in the 'night', in the darkness of unconsciousness, our self-awareness is born, just as the Holy Child was born in a manger, among animals, in the 'night', in darkness... He alone can reach God who has become thoroughly familiar with sexuality and tested it and all its potentialities to the full, either in this life or a previous one." (Haich 1982, 54-55) Sexual energy is the bearer of life and God will remain beyond the reach of a person who is ignorant of sexuality. Full experience of sex can release one from its bondage and then the individual can exercise control over it and use it as a *creative power.*

Elisabeth observed that a person cannot serve two masters. One can direct the creative powers either to the higher or to the lower centers, not to both at the same time. It means that there is a stage at which the individual stops the use of lower centres and, from then on, only higher centres are concentrated upon. By this time, sexual desire has fallen away from the person like a ripe fruit from a tree. Although the sexual organs are strong and healthy like in any other normal person, the potency goes into a dormant state with respect to them. Their energy is spiritualised and it is used only in the divine creative way. Truly great persons have never lived licentiously and they have been way-showers to others on the path of liberation. These ideas are corroborated with the teachings of Master Pythagoras, who used the symbol to say that one can either go on the path of spirituality or on the path of worldliness, but not on both at the same time. The fact is further confirmed with the traditionally old Hindu teachings. However, it is difficult to find the liberated people, since from the outer appearance they look the same as others. They are mainly recognised by those who are just below the level of the saintly person.

Among several researchers, in recent years Barabara Harris Whitfield is the one who, after journeying herself from sex to spirituality and after interviewing several men and women who had successful experiences, has written the book *Spiritual Awakenings*. According to her, spirituality and sexuality are the two sides of one coin, the coin being our nature. Sexuality is the doorway to higher realms of transcendent consciousness. People confided in her that their spiritual awakening happened during lovemaking and was preceded by the rush of Divine Energy. Some participants and speakers told her of periods in their journey where they wanted celibacy. The timespan she has heard, and practised herself, is a year or two. For some it becomes a permanent choice. Barabara observes that the path of intimate relationship may not be for everyone. It may even be inappropriate for some or in some situations. "Divine Energy makes itself known personally. Two then understand and experience the sacred three (God, you and me) becoming one... union with God is a direct personal experience. Sexuality connects us into a frequency of ecstasy that then connects us back to our Divine Source." (Whitfield 1995, 135) According to psychoanalyst and natural scientist Wilhelm Reich, making love is humankind's attempt to return to the original, unimpeded flow of cosmic energy. Barabara opines that the blissful moment involves three basic elements: transcendence of time, transendence of ego and being totally natural. These three things which give us ecstasy, just happen in sex naturally. Once these three elements have been experienced in sex, one can experience them in meditation too, or vice versa.

According to Barbara, the science of sex cannot be grasped in a day. Yet, however, persistent efforts can bring results. Her method of *spiritual sex* is to prolong the act of coitus and remain in the relaxed state while connected genitally, similar to meditation. There should be no thrusting movements except when erection is being lost and then it should be gentle thrusting simply to maintain penetration; full erection is not necessary. The two partners should be at right angles so that the contact is purely genital. There should be no talking and the mind should only be used to sense that is happening. Just feel the flowing warmth, the flowing love and the energy in contact. There should be awareness, without strain and a feeling of effortless floating. In a short time, the valley appears, you have relaxed orgasm and transcendence happens. There is not sex any more but the meditation of peaceful ecstasy. Von Urban says that the energy cycle becomes apparent, and within 28 minutes, the bliss sets in and continues for a long time. Barbara's talks with others showed that it happens sooner and transcends time. Regular meditation and spiritual sex both last about 20 minutes. There is a feeling of being younger, livelier and renewal of energy. The key words are: tension, letting go and awareness.

In Chapter 2 of my previous book (Kumar 1998), I have elaborated upon the fact through a variety of examples that married persons have been more successful in their spiritual quest, in comparison with celibates. Cases are drawn both from East and West and from saints to average householders. Many people married more than once in order to find a suitable partner. It may be that "*Tantric* sex" has been used by people in one way or the other, knowingly or unknowingly.

Osho Rajneesh spent his whole life in perfecting the method of ecstasy, preaching it to others through several centres round the world and he wrote a large number of books on the subject. According to him, there is no deeper mystery, no deeper secret, no deeper subject than sex in the world and in life. An average person goes through the routine of coitus throughout his life without knowing what it is. Those souls are rare who understand fully the art of sex, have passed through intricacies of sex, have had a rich sex life in previous births, and are now in a position to attain to the stage of *real celibacy.* Sex has become useless for them and through perfect celibacy they can reveal the truth about sex and divinity. There are a few valuable observations he has made. The first point is about the period of coitus. An average person lasts for about a minute and will desire it again the next day. If the period can be prolonged to three minutes, one may not want it again for about a week. A prolongation to seven minutes may not need sex for three months and an extension to three hours may free a person for the whole life. Such a coitus is *samadhi* which results in contenment and bliss that lasts a lifetime. A perfect coitus leads to real *celibacy.* In an average person, this does not happen and one carries the passion of intercourse to a ripe old age without satisfaction. His suggestion is to make the breathing slow. The faster one breathes, the shorter one lasts in the intercourse. Deep breathing through *pranayama* is a way out. Regular practise can bring the stage of *sex-samadhi* which opens the door for *realisation.*

The second point is that during the act of intercourse one should focus the attention on the third eye, that is, at a point between the eyebrows. The duration of climax will thus be prolonged to a long period, even one to two hours or more, and a state of *samadhi* leading to *celibacy* can be achieved. No one can attain celibacy without a real experience of sex. A successful celibate in this life owes it to a deep coital union either earlier in this life or in a previous life. "If, during sex, one has had an absolute revelation, even once, he is released from sex for the unending journeys of lives." (Rajneesh n.d. 112)

The third point is to give a sacred status to sex in life. During coitus, one is close to God, and as such, one's attitude should be as that of a man going to a temple, a church or a mosque. If one approaches sex with a pure mind and with a feeling of reverence, one can get a glimpse of the Supreme. Sex is sublimated and bliss is achieved. According to Rajneesh, sex is the re-experience of the original unity. A glimpse of the Eternal will convince one that sensual pleasures are meaningless.

The steps to be followed in *spiritual coitus* can be summarised as follows:

i) Develop slow breathing to stay longer.
ii) Keep your awareness between the eyebrows.
iii) Have reverence for the Creator.
iv) Approach sex when you are cheerful, full of love and prayerful.

The temples at Khajuraho, displaying the art of sexism and eroticism, near Chhatarpur, Madhya Pradesh, are said to be built by the Chandela kings of medieval India. "Khajuraho temples are the juxtaposition of religion and sex. Erotic sculptures on the walls of the Khajuraho temples have religious sanctity and philosophical background." (Dey n.d. 38-40) According to Dey, it symbolises *yoga* (divine unity) through *bhoga* (worldly pleasures). *Tantric* scholar, Sir John Woodroffe, says, "The practitioner is taught not to think that we are one with the divine in liberation only, but here and now, in every act we do, for in truth all soul is *Shakti*. It is Shiva, who as *Shakti*, is acting through the Practitioner. When this is realised in every natural function, then, each exercise thereof ceases to be a mere animal act and becomes a religious rite–a *yajna*. Every function is a part of the Divine Action in Nature." The *Brihadarnyaka Upanishad* states in a couplet, "In the embrace of his beloved, a man forgets the whole world – everything within and without, in the very same way, he who embraces the Self knows neither within nor without."

My Observations: The way from sex to Self/God is straight and short but not so easy. It might take several years or even more than a lifetime unless the method is understood and applied properly. And, of course, there have been innumerable people who have achieved success in a single lifetime. I would say that sex, combined with yogic practices and concentration between the eyebrows, which prolongs the duration beyond belief, and with reverence to God, can bring freedom from sex on one hand and Self-realisation on the other, within few years in a single lifetime. This has been my way and I have called it *regulated sex.* (Kumar 1998) This is *tantric* sex and has also been professed by Osho Rajneesh, as discussed earlier. However, there is another way suggested by Barbara Whitfield through which she achieved success. And, of course, there would be other techniques practised by people over the millenniums.

The stage of "freedom from sex" is clearly known by the practitioner through dreams, visions and direct feelings. For example, one may see in dreams that one's sexual organ is separated from the body like a ripe fruit and the person is putting it in some place in the house. Although he may still desire the company of the opposite sex, yet there is the difference of earth and sky. It may be for convenience and for the propagation of the teachings and not for sex as before. In fact, if only one of the partners is on the path to God, the other partner begins to complain about the irregularity of sex since he/she still needs it as before.

Self-realisation just happens without warning; one may be in the midst of coitus or doing some routine work or otherwise. One begins to hear the unstruck sound through inner ears and see divine light through inner eyes. One witnesses the soul and manifestations of God in many different ways. One may continue to live – eating, drinking, wearing clothes, travelling, etc. – as before, but the inner transformation has taken place. The person may not be recognised as such from outside because he appears similar to others.

I would further include disciplines from other branches of yoga to make the process foolproof, as far as possible. This would be the subject matter of the next chapter.

The geniuses in the past used to design methods through which the inner reality could be shown by outer physical symbols for the understanding of the common person. For example, the seven *chakras*, which exist in abstract form on the spine of a human being, have been shown as temples on the Himalayan range, beginning from the temple of Kamakhya Devi in Assam, to the temple of Vaishno Devi in Jammu and ending at the Amarnath temple in Kashmir. Similarly, the inner reality of God-realisation, which is achieved after the annihilation of sex, is shown in the temples of Khajuraho where one sees erotic scenes on the walls outside and the image of God inside the temple. Should not mankind pay great regards and thanks to these geniuses?

There has always been a controversy regarding sex after liberation. It is correct that truly great men have never lived licentiously. Those who have achieved a very high spiritual level and still have sex, although on rare occasions, have not yet become *whole*; they are on the path of becoming *whole*. Another view, however, is that if a saintly person once had a physical union with his loved one out of true love, with inner devotion and a healthy physical desire, he should not be considered on any account to be either a weak, fallen or a sinful person. After transformation of the energy, one experiences the union of "I" and *Logos* or *Om* and through "faith and surrender" one lives under the control and direction of the Spirit, having given up self-will. The same Spirit may some time direct one to have a physical contact with one's beloved, although the *two may be living as celibates normally*. After all, even sex is a manifestation of the Spirit.

Other Methods

Prayer is yet another way of opening oneself to higher consciousness. The results may vary from passing an examination to a direct experience of God, depending on the intentions of the person and intensity of the prayer. Visions appear to persons, especially to those who have already evolved through one or the other method, and open the gate to a higher or cosmic consciousness.

Emotional intensity is very high during moments of grief, joy, fear, gratitude, loss and so on. At such moments, repetition of a memorised prayer, or otherwise, a sincere request made to God through any kind of words is known to be heard in several cases. One feels connected to a Power receiving a sort of communication and security, and finds oneself in a reality beyond the physical with an abundance of peace and happiness.

Muslims advocate special prayers five times a day so as to maintain a connection with Allah. There are people with a religious bent of mind in all religions and sects, who keep remembering God through constant prayers throughout the day and remain in a state of exalted happiness and security, almost disconnected with the material world. And to touch the height of what a sincere prayer can do, let me narrate the following happening from ancient India:

There was a boy in a poor family who used to go to school in a neighbouring village. One day, he complained to his mother that all other boys arrived with a security guard to leave them to and take home from school every day. That very day, there was a party in the school in the evening and the boy felt afraid of crossing the jungle in the dark. He requested his mother to arrange a guard for him. Needless to say, the mother could not do it since they were poor. But she told the boy that his brother Kanhaiya (another name for Lord Krishna) lived in the very jungle he used to pass through. Whenever he felt afraid of something, he could call for Kanhaiya sincerely and loudly and Kanhaiya would immediately come to his help. The boy believed his mother completely and called for Kanhaiya that evening while going to school. And lo! there was Kanhaiya, clad in the traditional dress of that time and holding the flute in one hand. The boy caught a finger of Kanhaiya who led him to the school safely. On the way, the boy asked Kanhaiya for a small glass of milk he wanted to carry to the school as his contribution. Kanhaiya gave him that too.

The boy entered the school happily and handed over the glass to the man in the kitchen. After a while, as the boy was enjoying the function with others, the headmaster came running to the boy and asked him about the person who gave him the glass, since the milk in it, never got depleted however much he poured the milk from it into the big container. The boy told everyone about Kanhaiya and said that He would come to fetch him at the end of the function. Everyone waited for that moment, and when Kanhaiya came to escort the boy, only the boy could see Him and no one else. The boy was smiling and describing the clothes Kanhaiya was wearing, the flute He was carrying, the peacock feather He was wearing in his hair, and so on. But no one could get a glimpse of Kanhaiya in spite of their best efforts. On reaching home, he told everything to his poor mother who could make out what had happened and she thanked Lord Krishna from the crore of her heart, although she too could not see Him. He is visible to the pure, innocent and the devoted. Our so-called intelligent people with many professional degrees and a lot of wealth can easily disbelieve the truth of the happening, but there are those who believe it cent per cent. One is referred to the book *From Sweeper to Saint* by Baba Haridass (1980); the book contains about ten such real instances from India. Baba Haridass is presently the Chief Monk at the Mount Madonna Yoga Centre near Santa Cruz in California.

Freedom from Choice is a state of being which "Krishna called *Moksha,* that Jesus called Kingdom of God, that Buddha called *Shunyata* (Void), that J. Krishnamurti called Choiceless Awareness, the Awakening of Intelligence". (Jayaram 1997, 10) According to him, it is in that equanimity that the silent lake of our consciousness reflects the majesty of our amazingly intelligent universe. The situation can be understood through a Sufi story as follows:

There were two friends; one of them always maintained good health, while the other one grew weaker and weaker every day, until one day he reached the deathbed. The healthy one always used to eat his food from one bowl, irrespective of the different taste of its different ingredients. The other one used to eat the sweet food from one bowl and the bitter one from the other. On his deathbed, the one defeated in life, asked his healthy freind to tell him the secret of his good health. His friend answered that he would simply eat all the food from just one bowl, without making any distinction between the sweet and bitter eatables. On being pursued, the weaker friend ate, for the first time, all his food from one bowl and he felt a little better. Then, he started eating all his meals in one bowl. To the amazement of all, he soon recovered his health and began to live a healthy and normal life.

Truth is one, beyond all kinds of dualities, such as good and evil. It is "totality" and its division into fragments, such as associating oneself with one religion or sect or race, leads to disintegration which results in disliking and fighting with each other. This identification motivates the phenomenal "self" to become our master and the real unifying "Self" is pushed behind. Choice divides, division leads to conflicts. A confused mind chooses between this and that. A clear mind eats everything from one bowl and in that equanimity there is no struggle, no disease. In equanimity, the Self is realised.

As we know it, equanimity is the result of Self-realisation. Can the converse be made true, that is, can we cultivate equanimity in life and arrive at Self-realisation? If yes, this is a way to higher consciousness.

God-less "Karma" is another way to achieve higher consciousness and salvation, as it is advocated by "Jainism", the sixth largest religious group in India, after the Hindus, Muslims, Christians, Sikhs and Buddhists. It is an atheistic religion which has no room for God as creator-controller-destroyer of the universe. There is no agency to award favours and punishment; the doctrine is an automatically functioning mechanism. It stresses the supremacy of moral law. No prayers and worship are of any avail against the force of the *karma.* (Jain 1997, 12)

Whether a monk or a householder, a balanced individuality can be cultivated through the subjugation of passions like *krodha* (anger), *maana* (pride), *maya* (deceit), and *lobha* (greed). Renunciation consists in doing away with love and hate. Beyond *dukha* (misery, pain or suffering) and *sukha* (comfort, happiness) is *nirvana* or *moksha* (eternal bliss, emancipation, salvation), which is the true happiness and ultimate goal of the *atman.* True happiness results from the destruction of all *karmas* and cultivation of right conduct (*Samyak-charitra*), which is based on right belief (*Samyak-darshana*) and the right knowledge (*Samyak-Jnana*). The ethical discipline (*Achar dharma*) is prescribed for the fourfold community consisting of *sadhu* (monk), *sadhvi* (nun), *sravaka* (layman) and *sravika* (laywoman). The five vows to be taken by a disciple and to be followed rigorously are *Pranatipata Viramana* (to desist from killing), *Mirsavda Viramana* (to desist form telling a lie), *Adattadana Viramana* (to accept not when not rightly bestowed), *Maithuna Viramana* (to desist from sex), *Parigraha parimana* (to fix the size of acquisition).

Meditation deserves to be a separate article in itself because of its overwhelming importance, having been recognised the world over. But there are a large number of ways in which meditation can be performed and different systems of self-realisation adopt different techniques. For example, in Zen, as well as in *Vipassana,* the focus is on the breath, watching exhalation and inhalation passively, until the meditator becomes the breath itself – a relaxed mental flow being established wherein there is no one breathing and no one watching. Thus *kundalini-yoga* has its own way of meditation, which we are going to explore in a greater detail in the next chapter.

At the lower level, a variety of meditative techniques are used simply as a way to increase awareness, which is threatened in our contemporary world of speed and mechanisation. There are professionals who use meditation as a tool to help them manage stress or to increase their capacity for sustained work or to maintain general good health. Being centered, one feels free from frustrations and concerns.

At the higher level, it is the art to "look within" which leads to cosmic consciousness and Self-realisation. The word Buddha has become synonymus with meditation over the last twenty-five centuries. He achieved a hat trick by being born, enlightened and passing away on the same day, that is, May 11. Buddha used two words which are relevant in the modern context of one-sided development – sight and insight. "Sight with insight is wisdom. It is the bridge which conducts one's life to the ultimate truth. Buddha says that the main, if not the only, means to get insight is through meditation." (Wangchug 1998, 12)

Dr. A. Kasamatsu and Dr. Hirai conducted an experiment on Zen masters and pupils in 1960s. Preponderance of alpha waves, with some rhythmical theta waves as well, was found to be developed by the monks during meditation. "Alpha brain-waves run 8 to 13 cycles per second and are connected with a relaxed yet alert mental state. Theta waves run slower, 4 to 8 cycles per second and are generally related to a state of drowsiness, creativity, and the dream part of the sleep cycle." (Dalal 1998, 12) Decrease in the rate of respiration, a slowing down of the heart, lowering of blood pressure and a reduction in the need of oxygen were some of the effects of meditation, as found by researchers at Harvard and California universities.

Regular and systematic practice of meditation for twenty to thirty minutes a day is the key to success. In three to five years, people start reporting experiences. Out-of-body experience, in which one views one's body from a vantage point in the room, feeling of expansion that one has become larger, coinciding with the universe, visions of galaxies and stars, and writings in Hebrew, Latin or Sanskrit language for teaching the practitioner are some of the common experiences. Barbara Harris Whitfield (1995, 4) used to hear her own chuckling and the sound seemed to reverberate throughout the universe.

Guided meditation or *creative thinking* is also used to achieve higher states of awareness. As an example, imagine yourself sitting in a dark cave. You are bound by chains so that you are not able to move. Feel that a ray of light is coming from somewhere and is now suddenly falling on you. With this, you get the power to stand up and walk towards the opening of the cave and slowly you are out of the cave. You find that there is light everywhere and you are full of energy. You suddenly raise your hands and shake your whole body with great strength. One by one the chains break down and you are now free. You exclaim with joy and happiness and speak loudly, "I am a free person; nothing can bind me now, and I can do whatever I like."

As another exercise, imagine that in front of you there is a big statue which is sitting cross-legged. Look at the face, you find that it is you. Now imagine that your Guru appears on the scene with a spade. He tries to move you with his bare hand but he cannot since you are firmly rooted to the ground. Then, he puts the spade between your body and the ground and applies pressure to raise you up. He does not succeed. An associate of your Guru now arrives with another spade and applies pressure form the other side, along with your Guru on one side. Both of them keep trying for some time but you are so firmly grounded that they do not succeed. After some rest, the two senior persons try again to raise your statue up from the ground and with great efforts they are successful in raising it up slowly. Like two weightlifters, they bring the statue up to their shoulder level and put it on their shoulders. Both of them are now smiling and you notice that you are smiling as well. Slowly, both of them carry the statue towards a raised platform and put it up there. The statue gets life into it, stands up and raises both of its hands up towards the sky with a smiling face.

With a regular practise through exercises of this kind about an hour every day, you are likely to find your consciousness raised up in due course. This is an aid to Self-realisation.

Zen might be called the inner art and design of the East, taken to China by Bodhidharman from India in the sixth century. From there, it went to Japan around the twelfth century. Zen has been described as "a special teaching without scriptures, beyond words and letters, pointing to the mind essence of man, seeing directly into one's nature, attaining enlightenment." (V. N. N. 1998, 12)

Martial Art is more than just a means of self-defence or fighting. Says Kaicho Tadashi Nakamura, Grandmaster and founder of the World Seido Karate Organization, "Seido Karate is a way of life. It develops the spiritual being as much as the physical." Martial arts require a high degree commitment, dedication and self-discipline. "The practise of the martial arts also enables one to keep one's cool under pressure and to think clearly in the face of stiff competition, just like a manager needs to do. The daily structured application of the art improves the concentration through the practise of Zen meditation." (Agarwal 1997)

The Pilgrimage of Haj is considered to be the highest form of Islamic worship by Muslims. The rites of pilgrimage are called *Sha'air* (symbolic objects) in the *Quran.* They symbolically represent the life of Abraham and his progeny. "Different stages of their enactment of God's scheme are repeated symbolically in the rites of pilgrimage, making pilgrims feel at one with tradition of Abraham and his descendants." (Khan 1998, 12) Perhaps, this is the way to open the door of higher awareness for them.

A pilgrim leaves his home and sets off for the holy land nearing Mecca, to commemorate Abraham leaving his native land Iran for Hijaz; he then exchanges his tailored clothes for two unstitched sheets, comparable to the simple dress worn in the days of Abraham and Ishmael. On reaching Mecca, the pilgrim walks around the house of God to commemorate Abraham and Ishmael walking around the same House to solemnise the covenant they made with its Master. The pilgrim then walks seven times between the hills of Safa and Marwa in memory of Abraham's wife Hajra, who wandered between those two hills in search of water. This rite is called *Saee.* Abraham performed this by first readying himself to sacrifice his own son, then completed the sacrifice by slaughtering a ram, on the command of God. The pilgrim then stones the devil at Jamarat. The pilgrim keeps uttering the words, "Here I am at your service, Lord," throughout the pilgrimage. The holy journey culminates on the assembly of pilgrims at the plain of Arafat. At the end of this divine service, the pilgrims pledge before God to live their lives in the spirit of Haj.

Solitude, or to tread the unfrequented ways as Pythagoras preached, is the way to Self-discovery. The capacity to be alone is a measure of emotional maturity. "The capacity to be alone thus becomes linked with self-discovery and self-realisation; with becoming aware of one's deepest needs, feelings and impulses." (Storr 1988, 21) In the words of Edward Gibbon, "Conversation enriches the understanding, but *solitude is the school of genius;* and the uniformity of work denotes the hand of single artist."

There appear to be two opposite poles of nature. The life of a normal or average person revolves round the hub of intimate relationships. The chief, if not the only, source of human happiness appears to be interpersonal relationships of an intimate kind, more especially the ones with sexual fulfilment. Nonetheless, the way of living of the creative individuals seems to run counter to this assumption. For example, "Many of the world's greatest thinkers have not reared families or formed close personal ties. This is true of Descartes, Newton, Locke, Pascal, Spinoza, Kant, Leibnitz, Schopenhaur, Nietzsche, Kierkegaard and Wittgenstein. Some of these men of genius had transient affairs with other men or women; others, like Newton, remained celibate. But none of them married, and most lived alone for the greater part of their lives." (Stor 1988, ix)

According to Graham Wallas, a sort of re-ordering process takes place in the brain during creativity, which he called *incubation.* A creative person develops some interest in a particular subject, gathers all connecting material and studies every possible thing related to it. He calls this first stage as *preparation.* After some time, the accumulated material reaches a boiling point and *something un-understandable goes on during the period of incubation* which forms a prelude to the next stage of *illumination.* It is in three stages – preparation, incubation and illumination – that the creative person receives a new insight and finds a solution to his problem, or one can order the accumulated material and put it under an all-embracing principle.

The great religious leaders have demonstrated the fact that solitude promotes insight and inner change; they retreated from the world and after illumination returned to share their revelation with others. Buddha reflected upon the human condition and meditated under the tree of Bodhisattava for about seven years which culminated in his enlightenment. According to the accounts of St. Matthew and St. Luke, Jesus spent forty days in the wilderness and then returned to the world to give his message. Mohammed used to withdraw from the world to the cave of Hera during the month of Ramadan every year. Anthony Storr has noted that St. Catherine of Siena spent three years in seclusion in her little room in the Via Benincasa during which she underwent a series of mystical experiences, before entering upon an active life of teaching and preaching.

Anthony Storr has collected information, according to which many noted philosophers and writers produced their best work in solitude of some kind or the other. Roman Philosopher Boethius was imprisoned in Pavia by Ostrogothic king Theodoric. He was tortured and put to death in about A.D. 525. While in prison, Boethius composed *The Consolation of Philosophy,* for which he is remembered today. Sir Thomas Moore, Henry VIII's Chancellor from 1529, was imprisoned in the Tower of

London, after which he was tried and executed in 1535. During imprisonment, he wrote the masterpiece of Christian wisdom known as *A Dialogue of Cumfort against Tribulation.* Sir Walter Raleigh was imprisoned in the Tower of London and after trial he was executed in 1618. During imprisonment, he wrote his famous work *The History of the World.* John Bunyan was committed to Bedford country jail in England from 1661 to 1672. During liberal conditions of imprisonment for twelve years, he wrote his spiritual biography, *Grace Abounding,* which was published in 1666. Also, a considerable part of *The Pilgrim's Progress* was composed during the same period. Dostoevsky spent four years in a prison camp since his arrest in 1849. During this period, his repressed memories were released and thereby he was relieved of his psychic blockages and morbid fixations. Although never alone in the prison, he was emotionally isolated and lacked companionship, which turned his attention inward and converted his dillusion with peasantry into mystical belief. Pen and paper being not allowed to him, he kept on writing his notebook, which resulted in the book *House of the Dead,* describing his experiences of the prison camp.

A perverse imagination of Marquis de Sade flourished in captivity; he eventually died in 1814 while confined in the asylum at Charenton. His famous works, *Justine* and *Journees de Sodome* were written in the fortresses of Vincennes and Bastille. Adolf Hitler dictated his *Mein Kampf* to Rudolf Hess while in prison for nine months after the failure of his *Putsch* in Munich. In his own words, "Without my imprisonment, *Mein Kampf* would never have been written. That period gave me the chance of deepening various notions for which I then had only an instinctive feeling." (Storr 1988, 60) Anthony Grey in

China and Arthur Koestler in Spain were put to solitary confinement; their experiences were televised and transcripts were published in *Kaleidoscope* by Koestler. Both men admitted that solitude triggered their feelings of symapthy for their fellowmen and they found themselves in touch with some kind of higher order of reality. They felt the abstract existence of something which cannot be defined or expressed. Anthony Grey found a new awareness and Koeslter got a feeling of inner freedom in which he confronted with the ultimate realities. On being shown the picture of a lotus growing in mud by a Chinese friend, Grey felt that a glimpse of heaven can be had in hell too. It is timely to comment here that Jawahrlal Nehru, the first prime minister of India, wrote *The Discovery of India* while he was in prison; and, Sri Aurobindo studied the *Bhagavad Gita* in prison, where he had repeated visions of Lord Krishna as a result of his meditation.

I can recall the events of my whole life in which I was repeatedly thrown into aloneness or solitude by some design of the nature. While I was less than a year old, my mother went for her studies in another town and I was left in the care of my grandmother. I used to weep due to separation from my mother. All my education from nursery to Master's degree was away from the family, for one reason or another, and I used to weep in loneliness. Coming to the professional life, I was mostly away from my wife and other family members for several reasons and I used to suffer from depression many times. I have served in eight countries and I have mostly lived by myself; many times loneliness biting like anything and I used to feel like striking my head against the wall. Nevertheless, it is in these later years of loneliness that I took to meditation and reading of scriptures seriously and I got experiences with the Spirit. Self-realisation and writing of several psychical papers and books is a boon of this aloneness. Until the prime of my life, I used to accuse solitude but later I had all praise for it. Perhaps, it is in solitude that the inner self grows to become the eternal Self.

Remarks

There are yet other ways, such as music, dance, performance of certain rituals and so on which can take the individual on the path of higher consciousness. However, one may have to pick up a more strict discipline after a certain stage of development.

Various methods, described in this chapter, have not the same result of produce. Thus, Vedic methods comprising different forms of yoga and methods of dream, sex and meditation, for example, have the capacity to take the practitioner unto the end-state of liberation from falsehood, and Self-realisation. Methods like NDE and the ones described under the heading of "Crisis and Suffering", on the other hand, are such that they initiate the person on way to liberation by showing them a glimpse of the reality beyond the physical. The individual is then supposed to adopt a more rigorous discipline, such as metaphysics or meditation, to complete the journey.

As Jiddu Krishnamurti has said, no two persons in the world are the same as can be seen from the fact that no two persons have the same fingerprints. Accordingly, everyone has to choose his own path. Even two disciples of the same Guru would not have exactly the same approach. One has to choose a method according to one's nature and disposition.

Vedic methods introduced a fourth kind of yoga, called the *Hatha Yoga* which is the source of *Kundalini Yoga,* that is a balanced combination of various methods. It pre-supposes that the individual is not developed in any area (even if it is not so) and takes one to a fuller development an all-round personality. If one is on the crossroads to choose a method, I would suggest him to pick up the fast and foolproof method of *kundalini yoga,* which is the subject matter of the next chapter.

5
SECRETS OF KUNDALINI AWAKENING

Introduction

Chapter 1 of my previous book (Kumar 1998) was devoted to a working definition of *kundalini* and the seven *chakras*. To reiterate the basic point, "Some people could write inspiring prose or poetry and some could compose beautiful music, while others could not; some students could get very high marks in examinations with little time given to studies, while others, in spite of long hours given to studies, could score only poorly; some people could fight on the battlefield for days together, while others could not even do their normal work properly; some persons are known for wonderful discoveries and inventions, while others live mediocre lives and die unnoticed." In course of time, it was found that there was a special form of energy within every individual. In some persons, it was found to be dormant, in some it was slowly evolving, while in a few of them, it was fully awakened. Although this energy has infinite capabilities, it has no form or dimension, and consequently, it has been conceived in different manners under different names in various traditions of the world. Perhaps, the Hindus have the oldest records of naming this energy *kundalini* and it has been depicted in various physical forms for the understanding of the common people. Amongst all the methods available for the opening of the gateway to higher consciousness, it is the method of *kundalini* which is the most dependable and authentic one; and, it is the one which takes the practitioner to Self/God-realisation and even beyond.

To awaken the *kundalini,* one should first understand the "secret of awakening" and then look for the best method of achieving the result. At the time of fear, high emotional feelings, mental or physical excitement, danger of some kind or deep felt gratitude, etc., one overacts oneself beyond limits and later everybody is surprised with the use of "unusual energy" having come into action. For example, under fear or danger of life, people are found to run at a speed with which they could never run in normal life; they could even beat an Olympian racer. Where does this "unusual energy" come from? This "unusual energy" comes from the storehouse of "infinite energy" called *kundalini;* however, the event takes place only under "unusual circumstances". So, the secret lies in creating the "unusual circumstances" in safe and steady manner, which would eventually awaken the *kundalini* on a permanent basis.

There are two ways of creating the "unusual circumstances": one, through *shaktipat,* that is, receiving direct transmission of energy through a Guru or a realised soul who has an awakened *kundalini* himself/herself; two, by creating the circumstances by one's own indigenous efforts. Although the method of *shaktipat* appears to be the easiest and most of the people will be tempted by it, it has its own difficulties and limitations. The difficulty lies in finding the real Guru, and, more often than not, people have fallen into the hands of wrong persons and have wasted major parts of their lives in futile efforts. This is because real Gurus are rare and most people posing to be one are only imitating "guruhood" and commercialising it to meet their own ends. Secondly, one has to be prepared through proper discipline to receive direct transmission of energy. Unprepared persons are seen going to lunatic asylums or are found to have damaged their system, which is not easy to repair. Thirdly, it has been invariably seen that whenever a person is well-prepared to receive the transmission of energy, a real Guru appears before him at the right time. As such, one should not be looking for a Guru here and there and wasting time, rather one should adopt a proper discipline to prepare oneself.

Another fact is that the lasting effects are received through one's own energy, rather than through *shaktipat*. What happens within oneself is more important, basic and fundamental; it is one's own real wealth. World famous spiritual leader Osho Rajneesh observed, "*Shaktipat* will not add to your wealth, but it will certainly step up its capacity to grow. The effect of *shaktipat* is indirect, and therefore you need it time and again." (Osho 1997, 153-154) It is like a flash of lightning in which one gets a glimpse of the road one has to pass, and of the temple which is one's destination of the journey. But once is not enough, it is needed for the second time and for the third. One can reach without *shaktipat,* although it may take more time and one may reach late. None the less, one will certainly reach the goal. But *shaktipat* is a help indeed. I would suggest that one should prepare oneself with one's indigenous efforts and be ready to receive the direct transmission from a Guru, if and when there is a chance. And, above all, *shaktipat* can be requested and obtained successfully through the *divine presence* Itself. In any case, "indigenous efforts" are a must.

When we come to "indigenous efforts", we find that two kinds of religions have evolved throughout the world – one based on meditation and another based on prayer. Through prayer, one experiences God to be above, in the skies. Through meditation, one raises something up from within, believing that there is something asleep at our roots. So, it is the concept of above and below which makes the difference between prayer and meditation. Once again in the words of Osho, "...By and by, religions of prayer have been loosing ground and dying out. There is no future for them; they have no future whatsoever. And religions of meditation are daily growing in potentiality, and they have an enormous future before them." (Osho 1997, 188) In my previous book (Kumar 1998), I have devoted one full chapter to show that most religions of the world have been using practices similar to yoga and meditation under different names of their own, and *kundalini* energy has been at the root of almost all faiths as the common denominator to open the gate of higher consciousness. "...Difficulty is that every such school is not aware that others are doing the same thing in their own ways." (Osho 1997, 210) Thus, *yoga and meditation* are the real "indigenous efforts" to create the "unusual circumstances" to awaken the "infinite energy" called *kundalini*. A scientific combination of all yogic methods is called by me "The Integral Path", which is proposed to be the "shortest path" to awaken the *kundalini*.

The Integral Path

Vedic methods defined in the previous chapter were shown to have three main branches: *Bhakti yoga* (path of devotion), suited to the people whose heart predominates over their mind; *Jnana yoga* (path of wisdom), suited to the people whose mind predominates over their heart; and *Karma yoga* (path of selfless action), suited to the people whose heart and mind vibrate at the same level. There was a fourth category introduced in the medieval ages which was for those people in whom neither the heart nor the mind was developed enough to qualify for any of the above three methods, and that is, *Hatha yoga*. This branch of yoga became so important over the years that the word *yoga* meant only *Hatha yoga.* According to Dr. Rammurti Mishra, "Yoga is mastery of mind. It is a *process* of dehypnotism. Yoga presents a scientific way and methodical effort to attain perfection through the control of the elements of the physical, metaphysical and psychical natures." (Zemke 1996, 40) "All the yogic *asanas* and *mudras* follow the patterns of our mind's different states; and they are the results of countless experiments and experiences. ...After thousands of experiments, it was found which kind of *mudra* is formed in a particular state of mind. Then, the reverse process can also be worked out, in which you can attain to a particular state of mind by forming the *mudra* that corresponds with it." (Osho 1997, 207) Thus, the first step in IP (Integral Path) is to learn and perform yogic postures (*asanas* and *mudras*) which produce "peaceful and thoughtless state of mind" and "concentration at third eye, that is, the point midway between the eyebrows".

Breathing is another process which is associated with the state of mind. If one knows how one breathes in a state of silence, then one can create that state of mind by regulating one's breathing to the way which corresponds with silence. Having attained such a state of mind, it is not possible for a person to be angry or to entertain feelings of sex, etc. This is done through *pranayama* (deep breathing). To this, we add three locks: root lock (*mool-bandh*), navel lock (*uddayan-bandh*) and throat lock (*jalandhar-bandh*). These three locks are used to pressurise the *chakras* from root centre (*mooladhar*) to eyebrow centre (*ajna*), that is, from the first to the sixth energy centres. Thus, the sleeping *kundalini,* under the base of the spine, is hammered through the "double attack" of deep breathing and three locks, which eventually becomes one of the causes of its awakening. Hence, *pranayama* with *three locks* is the second step in IP.

Shashanka asana is a special yogic posture which regulates the breath in both the nostrils to equal frequency on one hand and reduces breathing to the minimum on the other. This brings mind almost to the null-state and in a position to slip into meditation easily. One may recollect that while one is sexually aroused one's breathing rises to the maximum. Meditation is the opposite state in which breathing is required to be minimum. Thus, *shashanka asana* is the third step in IP.

Chanting of Om (Aum) with concentration on the third eye is the final step in IP which forces *ajna chakra* (eyebrow centre) to open up on one hand, and prepares the individual to slip into meditation on the other.

With all this preparation, one is now ready to go into meditation.

To leave no stone unturned, and to make the process more effective and quick, the following four disciplines are added to it: (i) *prayer,* in which the factor of "faith and surrender" towards God is invoked and God is invited into oneself as Light and Sound; (ii) The element of *Jnana yoga* (path of knowledge) is used through the reading of scriptures and case histories of realised saints, so that the covers on ignorance are removed one by one; (iii) the element of *Bhakti yoga* (path of devotion) is used through the chanting of a *mantra,* so that *love* is developed towards God; and, (iv) the element of *Tantra yoga* is used through learning and adopting the method of *regulated sex* by married practitioners, which acts as a catalytic agent in the process and liberates the person from sex itself, which is the necessary step before Self-realisation. The first factor of prayer precedes meditation, while the latter three factors are to be used at other times during the period of twenty-four hours.

Integral Path, which is the way of life to be adopted by the practitioner, can be briefly summarised as the "daily routine" in the following way:

Elements of Integral Path

1) Two, hour workshop early in the morning, comprising
   - i) *Yogic exercises* for about 45 minutes.
   - ii) *Pranayama* with *three locks* for about 20 minutes.
   - iii) *Shashanka asana* for about 15 minutes.
   - iv) *Chanting of Om (Aum)* with concentration on third eye for about 15 minutes.
   - v) *Prayer-Shaktipat from Divine:* Closing all the doors of physical senses, invite white Light as the personification of God and feel it entering your body through the crown centre. Feel that it is hammering your *kundalini* and opening the seven *chakras,* one by one. Gradually, you will go into the state of *samadhi,* experiencing yourself as *atman* and merging with the *Absolute* in the ocean of bliss.
2) Two-hour reading of scriptures and case histories of realised persons (path of knowledge), any time of the day.
3) Two-hour chanting of a *mantra* selected by self or given by a Guru (path of devotion), any time of the day.
4) Married practitioners should learn the way of regulated sex life. This is an additional factor which expedites the whole process as a catalytic agent, and liberates the person from sex itself, which is a necessary step before Self-realisation.

I would like to comment on the incapability of the people in devoting six hours a day for God. To obtain a degree in engineering, medicine, accounting, etc., one has to devote a day-tight-life for about 5 or 6 years. God is not cheaper than a degree. If you remember God on a part-time basis or half-heartedly, He will also reveal Himself to you on a part-time basis or half-heartedly, which might take several lifetimes. In fact, we have been having part-time approach to God for innumerable lifetimes and nothing has happened yet. A formula is presented here which can bring liberation from further incarnations, if followed as suggested. Those who cannot devote six hours to God due to their involvements in the affairs of the world, they have not actually earned this privilege through their *karmas* in the past lives. They have yet to learn many lessons on the school of earth before they can devote necessary time in search of Self or God. However, there is always a way out if the determination is strong, and one can begin with one hour a day and increase the time gradually. It is the way of life which is practical for a common householder of today; one can awaken the *kundalini* and achieve Self-realisation in one lifetime, and that too, without the help of an external Guru or *shaktipat.* On awakening, *kundalini* takes the role of a Guru. In the words of Swami Vishnu Tirtha, "To a yogi She is, what Lord Krishna was to Arjuna, a guide and driver of his chariot on the battlefield of this worldly war for spirituality." (Tirtha 1993, 134)

This is the method which evolves the personality of the individual in an all-round manner: physical, mental, emotional and intuitional – producing an ideal person.

Details of the Method

(i) *Yogic exercises:* Postures given in the following figures are to be completed in about 45 minutes. One should inhale before the beginning of the asana and exhale slowly as one disengages oneself from it. The set of postures will produce calm, thoughtlessness and an automatic concentration on the third eye. It gives an all-round development of the physical body and sublimates sexual desire into pure love.

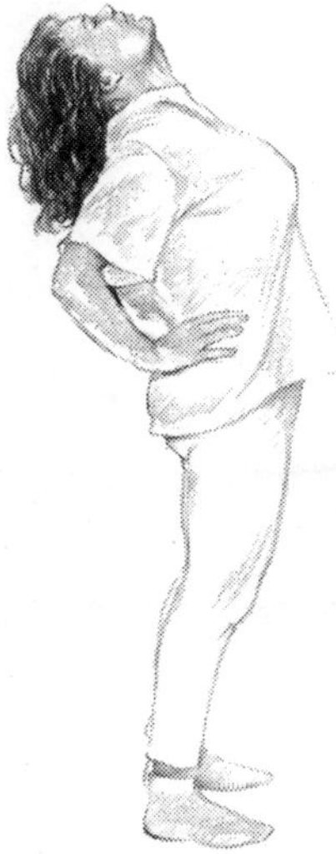

Stand straight with your feet about one foot apart. Keep your hands on the waist and bend backwards with eyes towards the sky. Do it six to ten times.

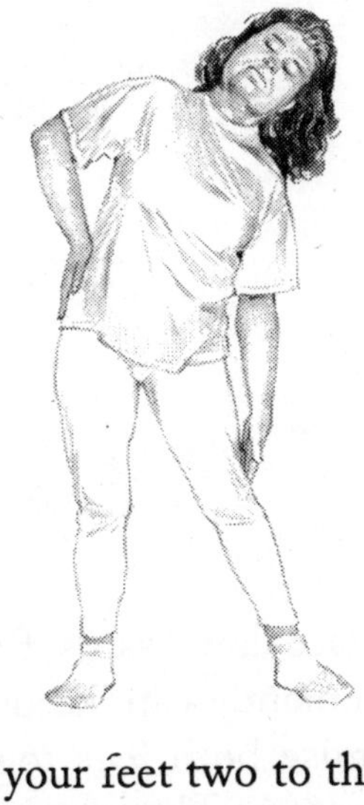

Stand straight with your feet two to three inches apart. Put your hands on your waist. Bend leftwards and touch your knee with left hand fingers twice. Do the same on the right side. This is one set. Do six to ten sets.

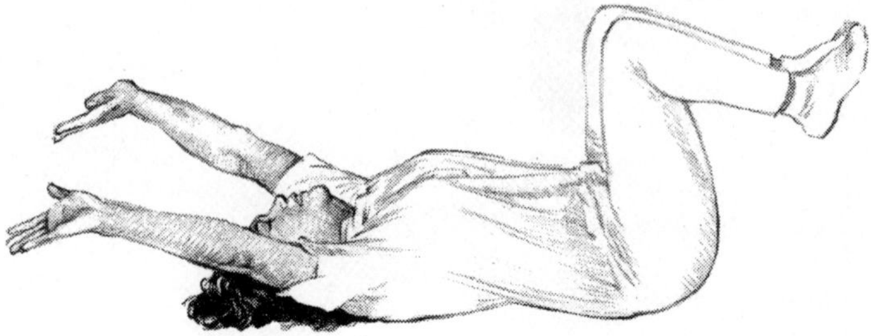

Lie down with your face upwards and yawn like a cat does, for some time.

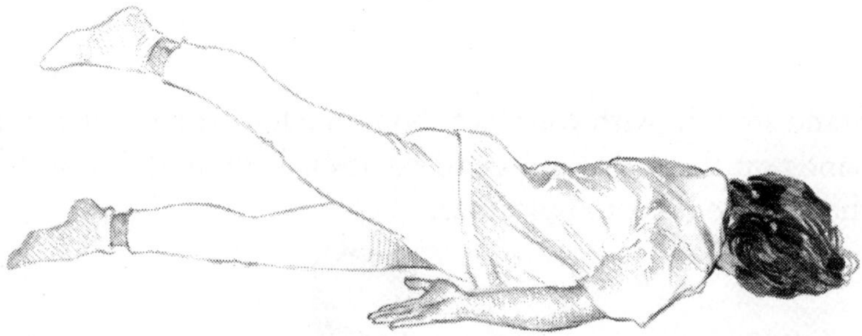

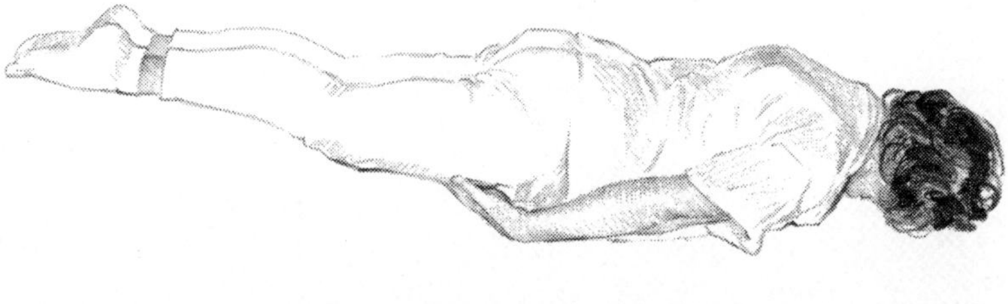

Lie down with your face downwards. Raise one leg at a time as high as you conveniently can, keeping it straight. Do it seven times. Now raise both legs together and hold the position for a few seconds. Then, lower them slowly to the resting position. Do it thrice.

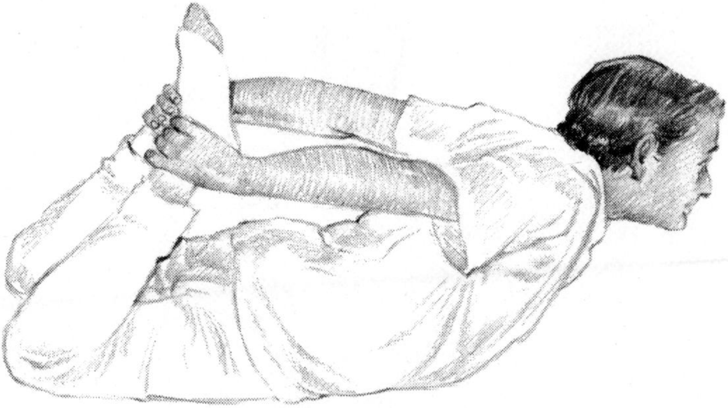

Bring your body in the position of a bow and hold it for half to one minut-

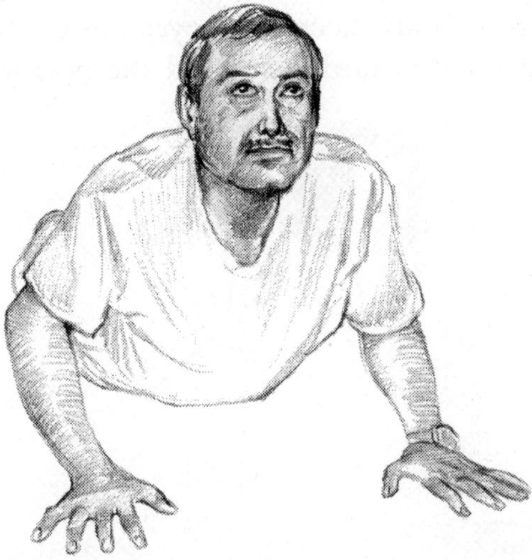

Bring your body in the shape of a cobra, touching ground with your navel region and turning your eyes towards the sky as much as possible. Hold the position for twenty seconds and do it two to three times.

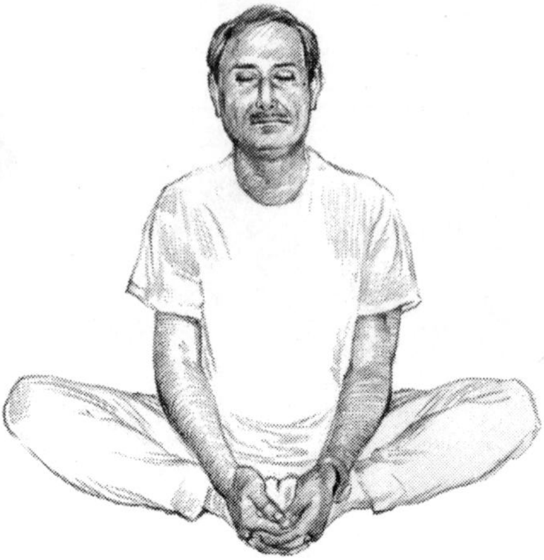

Sit straight, pulling your heels in with hands so as to press against your body, keep your eyes closed and focus your attention on the third eye. Hold the position for about a minute.

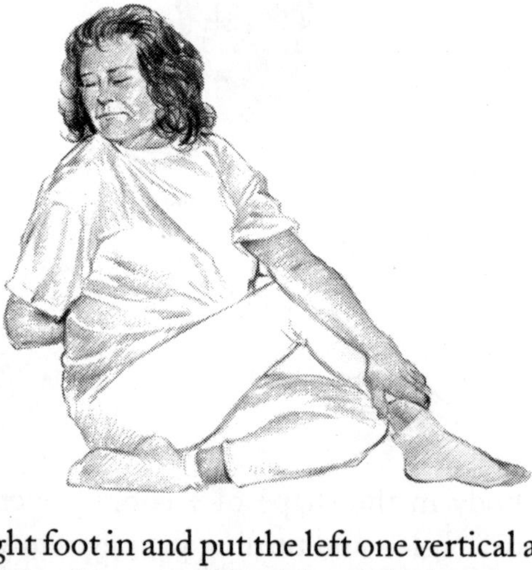

Turn the right foot in and put the left one vertical and touching the knee of the first one. Place the right hand across the left leg and hold the left foot with your right hand, twist the body towards the left as much as conveniently possible and look towards the left. Hold the position for twenty seconds. Repeat for the other side as well and hold for twenty seconds.

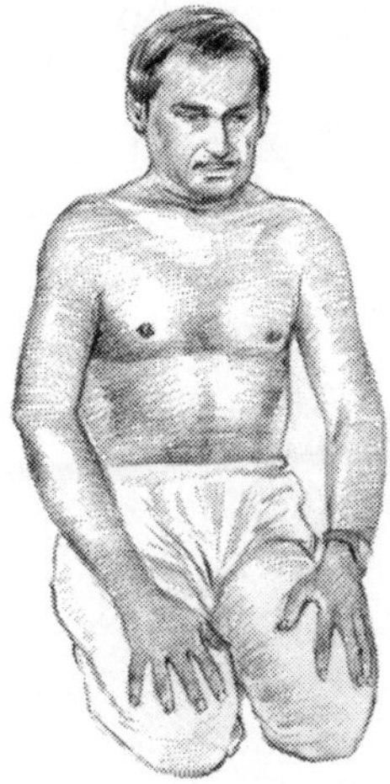

Sit on your knees with toes of both feet touching each other and heels apart, making room for your hips. Keep your spine straight, hands on your knees and attention focused on the third eye. Hold it for five minutes. Then breathe out completely and pull your stomach in and out alternately for about twenty to thirty times. Repeat the exercise four to eight times. This is perhaps the only pose which can also be held for fifteen to twenty minutes soon after eating a meal, to produce quick digestion. This is known as *Vajrasana.*

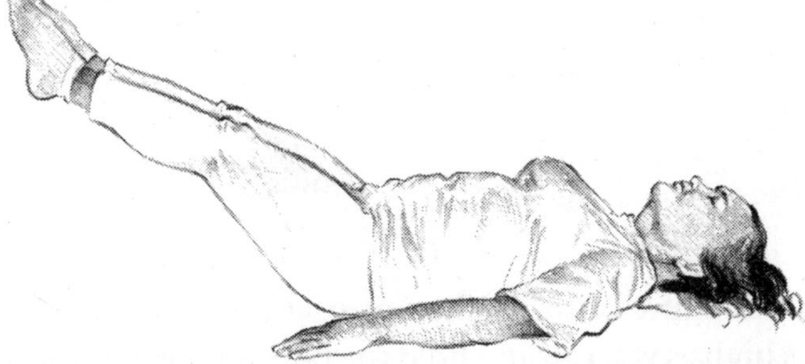

Lie down on your back. Raise one leg and hold it at an angle of 45 degrees for a few seconds and then lower it down in a slow manner. Repeat the same exercise with the other leg.

Do it for seven times. Now raise both legs together and hold them at an angle of 45 degrees for a few seconds and lower them in a slow manner. Repeat thrice.

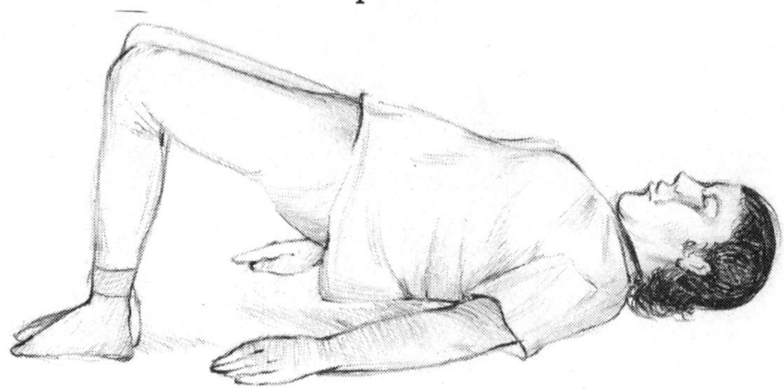

Lie down with knees bent and soles touching the ground. Raise your body from the middle, as high as you conveniently can, hold the position for about five seconds, then lower it down in a slow manner. Repeat the exercise seven to eight times.

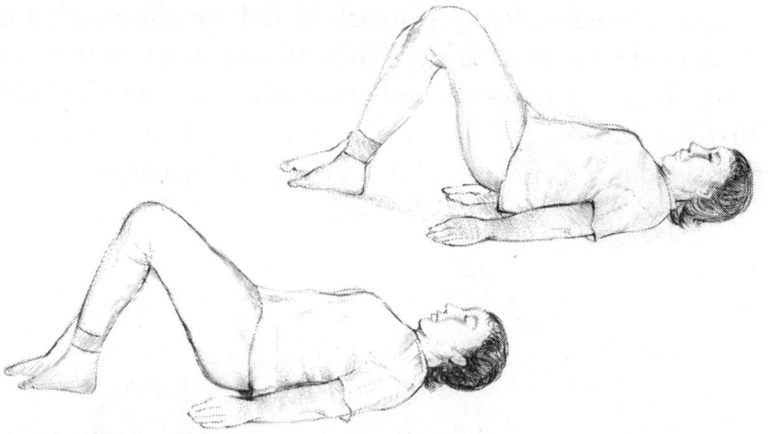

With the centre of the body touching the ground, raise your hips as high as you can and hold the position for a few seconds. Now, keeping the hips in touch with the ground, raise the centre of the body, making an arch for a few seconds, then lower down in a slow manner. Repeat the exercise seven to eight times.

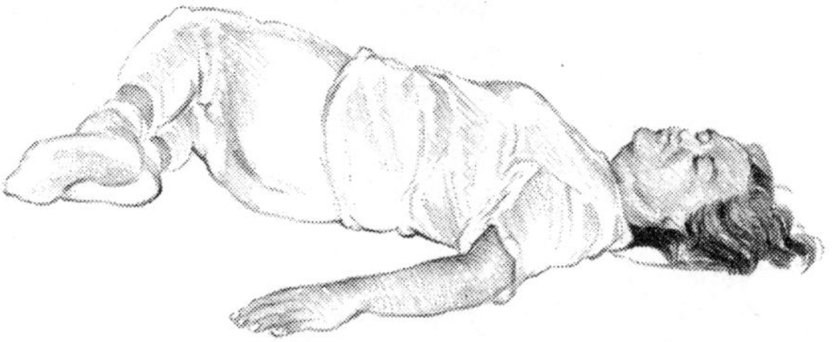

Lie down with knees bent and soles touching the ground. Move both feet together to one side till you touch the ground, keeping your face upwards, looking up at the sky. Hold the position for a few seconds, come to the original position and repeat the exercise, moving the legs to the other side. Repeat the exercise seven to eight times.

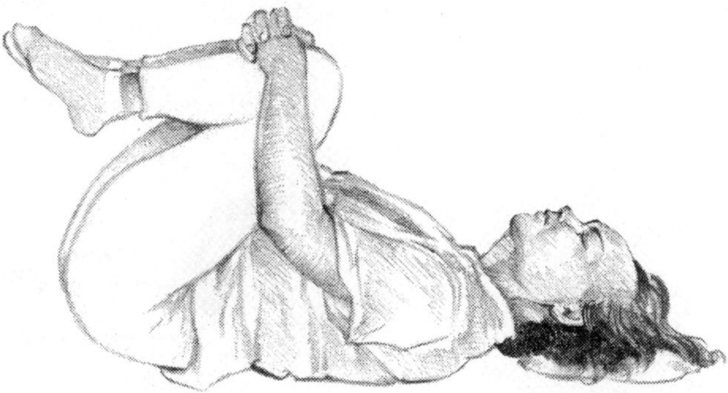

Lie down on your back. Bend the legs, hold them with hands and press them against your body twice, as closely as possible. This can be done ten times in two holdings of breath. Repeat the exercise with one leg, then the other, and then with both together once again.

After the set is complete, lie down on your back, hands and the whole body as relaxed as possible as if you are dead. Even thinking should be stopped as far as possible. This is to restore the blood circulation in the original position.

The following two postures are for *Pranayama*.

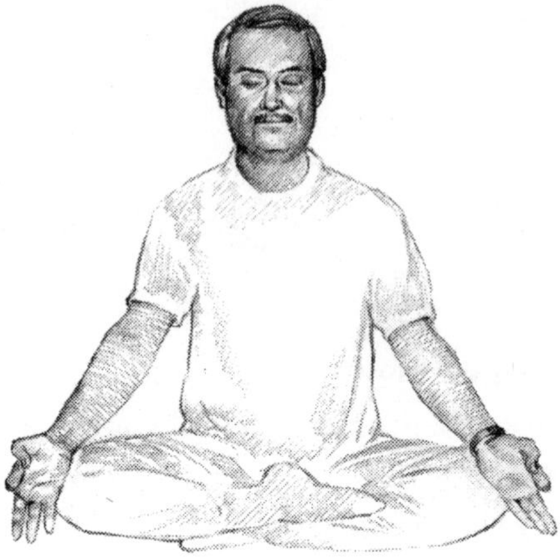

Siddhasana for men and *Siddhayoniasana* for women.

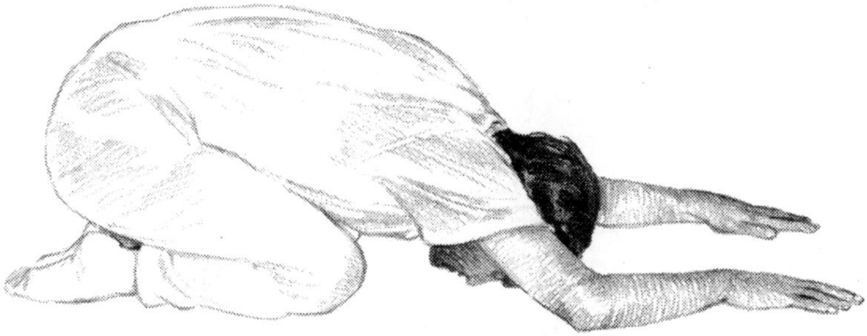

Sit in the posture of *vajrasana*, bend down to the ground with the head and nose touching the ground, and hands stretched out along the ground. Breathe naturally.

The two postures, *Shirshasana* (head-stand) and *Sarvangasana* (shoulder-stand) are very special yogic-postures, which are recommended for speedy spiritual growth, since they help in the reversal of the direction of flow of the seminal fluid. One can do either of them, depending on suitability, for any period, ranging from one minute to half-an-hour.

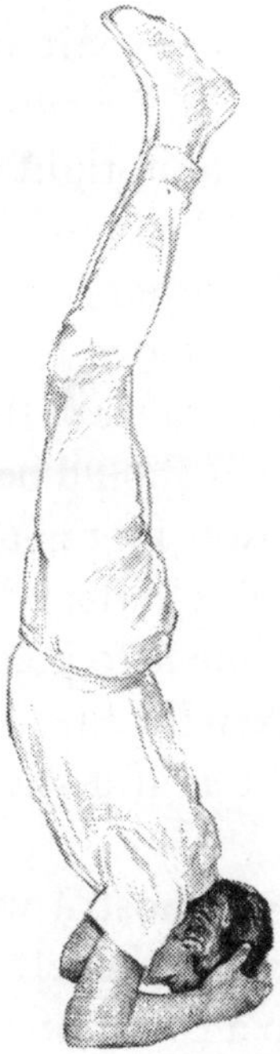

Shirshasana (head-stand)

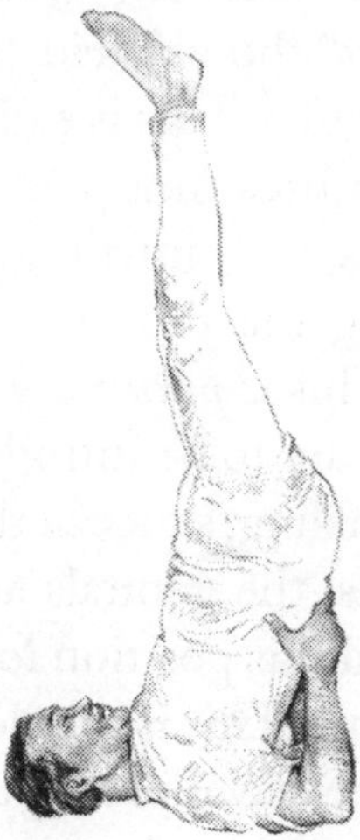

Sarvangasana (shoulder-stand)

(ii) *Pranayama* with *three locks:* Sit in the posture called *Siddhasana* (for men) and *Siddhayoniasana* (for women). In men, the heel of the lower foot, right or left, is to press the root centre (*mooladhara*) in the body under the reproductive organs and the heel of the other foot is to press the pelvic center (*swadhishthana*) just above the reproductive organs. Care should be taken not to squeeze the organs between the two heels and an adjustment should be made accordingly. In women, the heel of the lower foot is to be a little inside the vagina and to press that point in the body, and the heel of the other foot above the first one is to press the point just above the clitoris. This is to awaken the first two centres in the body. The spine will be straight as if a stick has been set in the ground.

Close the right (or left) nostril with the thumb of the right hand and inhale through the left nostril to a count of 4. Hold the breath inside to a count of 16. This is called inner *kumbhak*. Now close the left nostril with the small finger of the right hand and exhale slowly through the right nostril to a count of 8. Hold the exhaled position, closing both the nostrils, to a count of 8. This is called external *kumbhak*. This is one set of deep-breathing and the formula is 4-16-8-8. Repeat the process, now inhaling through the right nostril. Keep on repeating the process with alternate nostrils for twenty minutes. This is *pranayama*.

The *three locks* are to be introduced during *pranayama* as follows. While inhaling, squeeze the muscles of the anus and pull them upwards; the genitals are automatically pulled in and upwards. Hold this position for the complete duration of each set of breathing. This is root lock (*mool bandh*). Squeeze, simultaneously, the navel area, pull it inside and hold this position for the complete duration of each set of breathing. This is navel lock (*uddayan-bandh*). When inhaling is complete, at the count of 4, press the chin against the body and hold it for the complete duration of each deep-breathing. This is chin lock (*jalandhar bandh*). At the count of 16, when you begin exhaling, release all the three locks at the same time. *Pranayama* and the *three locks* are to hammer the sleeping *kundalini* forcing it to wake up, and pressurise the first five *chakras*, from the root to the throat, to open up. An automatic concentration on the third eye is produced.

(iii) *Shashanka asana:* Hold the posture shown in figure 16 for about fifteen minutes. You will find that the speed of breathing has slowed down considerably and you can easily slip into the state of meditation.

(iv) *Chanting of Om* with attention on the third eye for about fifteen minutes will bring tremendous concentration on the third eye which may result in the opening of the eyebrow centre (*ajna chakra*) raising the *kundalini* upwards and slipping into meditation. One should inhale fully and then chant Om till the breath lasts. You may sit either in *Siddhasana* or an easy posture or on a chair with your spine remaining straight. You should make yourself comfortable and well set since you are now ready to go into meditation.

(v) *Prayer-Shaktipat-Samadhi:* This is the final step of the two-hour workshop and you are well set to go in the state of meditation and one day you will just slip into *samadhi*, which is our final goal. Sit in an easy posture on the ground or on the chair with your spine straight, neither too tight nor too loose, just the right middle way. Close your eyes and keep your attention on the third eye. You are already in the state of calm and thoughtlessness, and ready to slip into meditation. Feel that you are sitting on this earth which is a globe and that you are rising up and up towards the Absolute. Feel that liquid white Light is pervading everywhere and you are feeling Its touch on every part of your body. And the same Light is filling your body from the crown centre to make your body immune to all kinds of decay, imperfections, diseases and accidents for the rest of life. Feel that the Light has accumulated in your root centre, pelvic centre, navel centre, heart centre, throat centre and eyebrow centre. All the *chakras* are open and are providing their full power to you. Mother *kundalini* has awakened from its seat below the spine and is rising through the spine and has reached the crown centre. You are enjoying the bliss and happiness of it. Nectar, in the form of white Light, is filling your head, then the neck, then the left shoulder and left hand, then the right shoulder and right hand. Feel that both your hands are longer and heavier than before because now they are filled with white Light. The Light is now filling your spinal column, the heart, the lungs, the kidneys, the stomach, the reproductive organs, the left leg and lastly the right leg. You are filled with Light and surrounded by Light; you have become Light yourself.

Liquid white Light is nothing but God Itself. You have received the *shaktipat* from God and you have become God yourself by His own blessings; because this is the only way. He is the ocean of love and mercy. He has forgiven all your faults, mistakes or sins, if any, and has burnt all your *karmas* through the awakening of Mother *Kundalini.* Feel that you are a pure being, an awareness other than the mind and body, feel that you are the dimensionless *atman* who is a witness to everything happening around. Feel that you as *atman* are rising up from physical to astral, mental, intuitional and soul plane and becoming one with the *Supersoul.* The drop is merging in the ocean and the ocean is merging in the drop. *Atman* and *Paramatma* have become one. Enjoy the bliss of the union and get lost in it. You are in *Samadhi.*

2) To meet the requirement of the *Jnana yoga* (path of wisdom), one should make it a habit to read the scriptures

and case histories of realised persons. This will quicken the process of awakening of *kundalini* through discernment of right and wrong and learning discrimination. The covers of ignorance will be removed one by one. I would recommend two hours a day, but it can be more or less, depending on several personal factors.

3) The requirement of *Bhakti yoga* (path of devotion) can be met through the chanting of a *mantra* which serves the double purpose of attracting spiritual energy from the cosmos and developing love for God. The process of *kundalini* awakening becomes faster. Thousands of years of research by several *yogis* and *rishis* has shown that the repetition of the names of God, even mechanically, bring the desired results. The mechanical process is gradually converted into reverence. Union of *atman* and *paramatma* becomes easy and smooth. As an example, one can pick up a simple mantra such as *Om Namah Shivaye.* The technique is to feel the beginning sound of *Om* to be emanating from the seat of *kundalini* and gradually rising upwards to the eyebrow centre with a pulling motion; the last two words *Namah Shivaye* to be spoken with a push into the position of the third eye. The *Sufis* have a very good technique of repeating the name of God which is similar to the one suggested here. In a conference during December 1996 in a Florida retreat, I came to know that one of the *mantras* that Lord Jesus used to chant was *Yod Hey Wod Hey* with a similar technique as above. In alchemy too, you have to chant a *mantra* to bring about the union of *Chang* and *Chi,* the male and female principles of the personality. As for the duration of chanting, I would again suggest two hours to get quick results, yet, it can be more or less, depending on the personal factors of the practitioner.

4) Last, but not the least, is the technique of *regulated sex,* to be learnt and used by the married practitioners. I have

shown, in my previous book (Kumar 1998), that most of the realised persons and yogis were married persons. However, they used sex for "generating an experience and sublimating it, opening, thereby, the doors of higher perception" rather than for sensual pleasure or procreation. Sex is a very important tool, if used properly. Just as a thorn in the body can be removed by a thorn only, even so, liberation from sex can be achieved through sex only. The technique has already been described earlier.

Comments

A single path can bring the desired results, nevertheless it is very difficult. For example, the path of selfless action (*karma yoga*) would require a person to live the life of Mahatma Gandhi or Mother Teresa, which is not so easy for a common householder. Similarly, the path of devotion (*bhakti yoga*) would require a person to be devoted in the service of God day and night like Mira, Surdas or St. Teresa of Avila. Path of knowledge (*jnana yoga*) would require a person to be studying about "truth" day and night like king Janaka, Ramana Maharshi, Richard Maurice Bucke, etc. Path of sex (*tantra yoga*) would require an individual to be engrossed in *tantric* rituals day and night. And then, there are chances for the practitioner to fail or to become eccentric since a single path would not develop the personality in an all-round manner. Hence, the researching yogis were led to develop a path which would combine the elements from various disciplines so that one could continue to live in the natural way and yet achieve liberation from the continuity of earthly incarnations. This gave birth to *kundalini yoga* and an Integral Path like the one presented here. Gautama Buddha taught the *middle way* between asceticism and rational living, and Sri Aurobindo advocated the Integral Path in his own way. The path presented here meets these requirements.

Sage Patanjali was the greatest exponent of yoga. The eightfold path advocated by him has the following steps: (1) *Yama,* meaning moral conduct, such as non-violence, non-stealing, truthfulness, continence and non-covetousness, (2) *Niyama,* meaning religious observances, such as purity of mind and body, contentment, self-discipline, study of scriptures and devotion to God, (3) *Asana,* meaning yogic postures, (4) *Pranayama,* deep breathing or breath control, (5) *Pratyahara,* meaning withdrawal of senses from external objects, (6) *Dharma,* meaning determination, (7) *Dhyana,* meaning meditation, and (8) *Samadhi,* meaning final absorption leading to oneness with the Supreme.

The Integral Path presented in this chapter happens to meet all the requirements of Patanjali in the modernised way, suiting the requirements of the present-day householders. Moreover, factors like *prayer* and *regulated sex* have been added for perfection and increased effectiveness.

The complete package of IP is, in fact, a way of life which is easy to adopt in a short time although it may appear difficult to look at. I found it very convenient while living the life of a university professor. And my feeling is that one can achieve results in a single lifetime, the period may vary from a few weeks to a few years, depending on how much one puts into it. However, there are certain yogic postures a particular practitioner may not like to do or a certain discipline one may not like to incorporate or one may put only two hours a day instead of six hours, yet, the person should go ahead and the progress is bound to take place, although it might take some more time to achieve the goal. And, with the advance of time, the missing factors may be added according to suitability.

The whole process can be understood well through the example of water. To boil water, you may have to arrange a few things and the fire should be powerful enough to bring the temperature of water to 100 degrees. All this may be cumbersome and time-consuming. But once the water reaches 100 degrees, it will not take it a second to convert into steam. Similarly, in yoga, you may have to make efforts of several kinds to bring yourself to the temperature of 100 degrees; and once this is done, manhood is converted into Godhood in no time. You may have to use several techniques and make sure that your self goes from 97 to 98, 99 and then 100 degrees, nothing short of it. And then you discontinue being a man, and begin to live as God. But remember that "there is always one step more". Godhood is an everlasting journey, from perfection to perfection. The only difference is that you have the satisfaction and bliss of being on the path and knowledge of the truth, while others live in ignorance, and material satisfaction is, for them, the beginning and end. You know that you have broken the cordon of further births, while others have to continue with the series of reincarnations till "that auspicious day" comes for them in a particular lifetime.

The Awakening of Kundalini

There are some characteristic symptoms through which the awakening of *kundalini* can be recognised; see, for example, *Kundalini – The Secret of Life* by Swami Muktananda (1979), *Mahayoga Vijnana* by Swami Yogananda, *Kundalini* by Ajit Mukherji or *The Serpent Power* by Sir John Woodroffe (1979). A comprehensive list of symptoms of the awakened *kundalini*, though not exhaustive, is presented here:

1) Throbbing of the root centre (*mooladhara*), shaking of the whole body, and involuntary inhaling and exhaling of breath with one's losing control of the body.
2) Trembling of the body, involuntary laughing or weeping, twisting of the tongue and deformed sounds coming from it, fear and frightening visions, standing of the hair on ends and secreting of semen.

3) Fixation of the posture and concentration between the eyebrows, revolving of the eyeballs and automatic holding of breath in the lungs (*kumbhak*), cessation of breath and creation of a void in the mind.
4) Fixation of the posture and involuntary coming of the three locks – root, navel and throat (*mool bandha, uddayan bandha* and *jalandhar bandha*), reverting back of the tongue and its rising towards the palate (*khechri mudra*), stretching out of hands and legs forcibly.
5) Feeling of the spiritual energy (*prana*) being active in your body day and night, concentration of mind fills the mind with joy and bliss and your body begins to shake or toss, and a feeling that the spiritual energy is rising to the crown centre every moment – whether you are attending to the call of nature, sleeping or dreaming.
6) Feeling that your mind and body are possessed by some Heavenly Agency or Spirit and under that influence your body performs involuntary yogic postures without any pain or fatigue and accompanied with some strange kind of breathing.
7) Hearing of different kinds of internal sounds (*naad* or *shabda*), feeling of absence of body and experience of vibrations in the spinal column, eyelids opening and closing without your efforts, a feeling of electrical currents passing through your nerves and you have convulsions.
8) Automatic repetition of *mantra* all the time, accompanied with the waves of blissful beatitude and passing of spiritual currents to the cerebrum.
9) The body possessed by some Heavenly Agency begins to rotate like a grinding stone, you lose control of breathing; sitting in a cross-legged position, your body

begins to jump like a frog here and there or the body becomes motionless like a dead person and you feel like passing away.

10) The moment you sit with your eyes closed, the body begins to throw limbs forcibly and you begin to utter deformed sounds or sounds (like those of various animals and birds).
11) Wherever you fix your attention in the body, the spiritual energy *prana* begins to flow there with your nerves undergoing jerks, as if electricity is passing through the wire.
12) Feeling intoxicated without taking any drug, walking like a drunk and unable to do any other work, your steps falling majestically, not interested in talking to or hearing others and a feeling of having drunk divinity.
13) Shaking of body and singing of hymns with joy and ecstasy whenever you sit for prayers, music and poetry coming out of you involuntarily, speaking languages you know not.
14) Maintaining balance of mind, undisturbed in all ups and downs, having acquired inexhaustible energy to work, not feeling tired even after many hours of work, feeling the body light like air, filled with joy and buoyancy and happy even in dreams.
15) While in meditation, you fall in a dreamy state of mind; divine visions, divine smells, divine sounds, divine tastes, divine figures, divine touches and divine instructions coming to you.
16) While in meditation, the secrets of future and hidden meanings of scriptures begin to unfold before you, removing all doubts; you begin to understand the spiritual works at a glance and acquire self-confidence

so that you do not feel the need of approaching anyone for knowledge, including Brahma himself, and you acquire strange powers of oratory and influencing the audience.

17) While in meditation, you get a quick concentration between the eyebrows, breathing slows down considerably and you plunge into the ocean of bliss, *khechari* and *shambhavi mudras* come into operation and you experience the pleasure of *savikalpa samadhi.*
18) Regularly in the mornings and evenings, you get charged with such divine influences and feel being possessed by a Heavenly Agency.

Comments

It is important to point out here that everyone does not get all the symptoms mentioned here. Only some of them will appear in each one, depending on the temperament and preparation of the individual. For example, if a person has been doing the necessary yogic postures as a part of his practice regularly, the involuntary postures will not manifest in him on awakening of the *kundalini*, since he has already met with those requirements. In a person, who has lived a natural sex life by way of his marriage, excessive heating of head or other parts of his body will never take place on awakening. Someone who has covered all the factors included in the IP, will have a very smooth awakening of one's *kundalini*, with none or very little side effects, and only positive symptoms will manifest in him.

Transformation and New Birth through *Nadis* and *Chakras*

The physiology of *kundalini* can be understood through its supporting elements – three *nadis* (subtle channels) and seven *chakras* (energy centres) – shown in figure 19. The connection of *chakras* with glands is shown in figure 20.

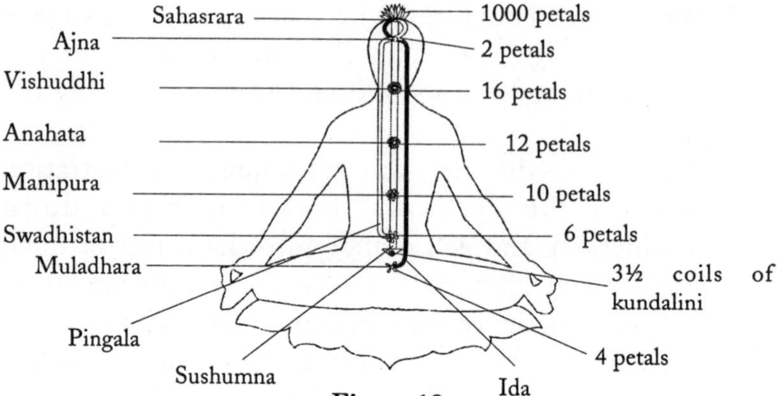

Figure 19

The three *nadis* are (i) *Ida,* (ii) *Pingala* and (iii) *Sushumna* – which create *chakras* (1) to (7) as shown in figure (19). The function of the *chakras* is to govern all aspects of our being and to supply energy to meet the basic needs. The seat of *kundalini* is at the base of the spine, between the first and second *chakras,* where it lies dormant in the form of a snake with three-and-a-half coils around the *swayambhu linga* and closing the opening of the linga with its mouth. The name *kundalini* is derived from *kunda*, meaning "cavity" in which it resides and, *kundala*, meaning "coils". The "feminine form" of the masculine *kundala* is *kundalini,* meaning thereby that this energy is recognised in the female form of "Mother". She is responsible for taking our attention to the highest level of realisation. She has an in-built archive which records all our previous existences, she has intelligence of her own, gives her loving care to us as the Mother and guides us in the best possible way.

Since *kundalini* is herself pure, she rises in a person who has achieved purity. On arousal, the anguish on the face of the practitioner changes into radiance; he begins to look younger, active, beautiful and magnetic. *Kundalini* repairs the damage, cures the illness and rejuvenates the body; and the

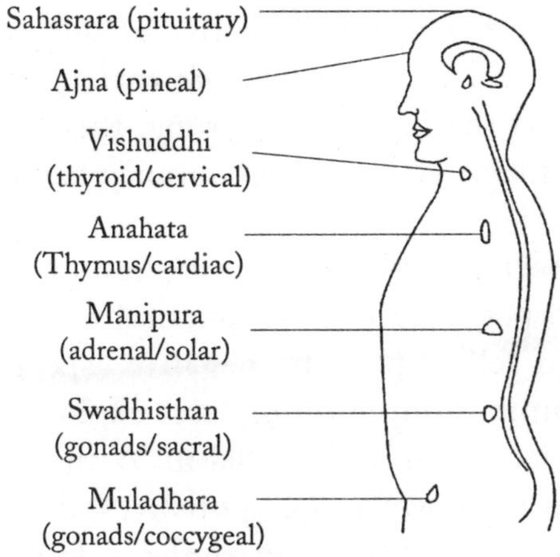

Figure 20

same sort of healing can be passed on to others by the successful practitioner. The power received is in direct proportion to the desire for and faith in *kundalini*.

The Nadis

In the set of three *nadis, ida* (moon channel) manifests at the left, *pingala* (sun channel) manifests at the right and *Sushumna* constitutes the central channel. *Ida* and *sushumna* begin at the *mooladhara chakra, pingala* begins at the *swadhishthan.* All of them cross at the *ajna chakra,* where *Ida* moves to the right and *pingala* moves to the left and the three nerves join again at the *sahasrara.*

Ida nadi represents *tamoguna* (inertia), the past and the subconscious. Its positive aspects are existence, emotion, joy, desire and auspiciousness. Its negative aspects are conditioning, superstition, lethargy, guilt, blind faith, self-pity, fear, day-dreaming, addictions, pornography, sexual perversion, blind faith and black magic. Since emotion is born out of desire, the left side of the body represents the emotional side. If the left side is weak, one becomes prone to emotional extremism, the negative aspects of the *nadi* are manifested and the growing pressure on the brain can lead to a breakdown;

in extreme cases, one may become epileptic, lunatic, etc. A balance should be achieved through *rajo-guna,* that is, activity of the right channel. If the left side is strong, the positive aspects of the *nadi* are manifested and joy, buoyancy, happiness are expressed.

Pingala nadi represents *rajo-guna* (activity, desire), future and supraconscious. Its positive aspects are physical and mental activity, creativity and self-respect. Its negative aspects are egotism, temper, domination, cunningness, exploitation, vanity, shamelessness, fanaticism and asceticism. With a strong right side, the person is known to be egotistic, selfish and aggressive and his emotional side may get paralysed. However, logic and wisdom in such persons are seen to depart soon and they are known to be stupids and idiots. A balance can be achieved by moving to the *sattva-guna* (purity) of the central channel *sushumna,* and believing strongly that "I am not the doer".

Sushumna nadi represents *sattva-guna* (purity), present and unconscious. It has only positive aspects, which are faith in religion, nourishment and revelation. It is the channel through which our evolution takes place. When partly active, it provides awareness, virtue and righteousness. *Kundalini,* on awakening, first ascends *sushumna* up to *ajna chakra,* and then descends through *ida* and *pingala* in a melting form. The disparate factors of our being begin to integrate in a whole. It connects the mind to the *atman.* Passing through the gate of *ajna chakra,* one reaches *sahasrara,* which is the Kingdom of God. Maintaining thoughtless awareness, meditation makes *sushumna* strong. One lives in "eternal now", transcending time and space.

Arousal of *kundalini* through *ida nadi* manifests negative aspects of *ida*, arousal through *pingala nadi* manifests negative aspects of *pingala*; it is only the arousal through *sushumna* which leads to the Kingdom of God.

The Chakras

Ripples are created by the respective powers of *ida* and *pingla nadis* in the two channels, and seven *chakras* are created at the points where these ripples meet. The *chakras* are vortices of energy, moving in the clockwise direction. Each *chakra* corresponds to a plexus and to a certain number of petals expressing its qualities. Each petal, in turn, corresponds to a sub-plexus. Seen from above, the chakras would appear as overlapping circles. They are storehouses of energy for the corresponding plexuses, meeting physical, mental, emotional and spiritual demands of the sympathetic nervous system. Before the awakening of the *kundalini,* the *chakras* have a limited and exhaustible energy, likened to a battery. After awakening, however, they are connected to the unlimited divine power-plant through the *kundalini* and then their energy is inexhaustible. These *chakras* evolve and develop at various stages and they represent the milestones on the path of evolution.

The first one is the *mooladhara chakra* (root centre) situated below the seat of *kundalini,* having four petals and earth as its element. Literally, *moola* means root, and *adhara* means support. This *chakra* represents innocence, eternal childhood, chastity, motherly love and wisdom. It is responsible for sex and excretion. Its negative aspects are adultery, perverted sex, pornography, lustful attention, materialism, no interest in spiritual quest and constipation. The Elephant God, Lord Ganesh is its presiding deity, who is known as the remover of obstacles, and the source of absolute wisdom. *After awakening, one achieves victory over sex, and one learns to develop respect for one's own chastity and that of others. A childlike mind goes through the process of maturing. Freedom from sin is achieved; sin in yogic terms is an intentional repetition of well-known mistakes, and so, it is in one's power to achieve freedom from sin. With the eradication of selfishness, one always lives in the spirit of gladness.*

The second one is the *swadhishthana chakra* (navel centre) suspended like a satellite on a chord from the *manipur chakra* (third), in the spine in the region just above the genitals, having six petals and fire as its element. The *kundalini* first awakens in the *manipur chakra,* passes enlightenment to the *swadhishthana chakra* through the chord and then returns to the *manipur chakra.* This *chakra* represents intellectuality, creativity, inspiration, knowledge of the beyond and aesthetics. It takes care of the kidneys, liver, spleen, pancreas and the uterus. Its negative aspects are excessive thinking and excessive involvement in artistic things, ego-oriented life – domination or slavery, alcohol, drugs, earning through talents, bad eating habits, artificial and crude behaviour. In positive sense, it bestows intelligence and creativity in conjunction with the *pingala nadi,* since its presiding deities are Lord Brahma and his power Sri Saraswati, the former being the creator and the latter being the goddess of music and arts. Since *pingala* draws its power from *sushumna,* an imbalance may be created, which may result in diseases like diabetes and heart attacks. A balance can be restored through non-materialism and non-egotism. Excessive thinking and attention can pressurise the liver. Interest in the knowledge of the dead or black magic are wrong pursuits which can damage the *chakra. One should aim at achieving the state of "thoughtless awareness"* (nirvichar samadhi) *and develop real humility. Increased awareness, ability of well-reasoned discourse or writing of prose or verse are the gifts of this* chakra. *Freedom from enemies – greed, lust, anger, attachment and ego – is achieved and one's mind dwells on the beauty of the Most High. The poet may touch the level of a prophet.*

The third one is the *manipur chakra* (navel centre) at the level of the solar plexus, having ten petals and water as its element. It represents righteousness, *dharma* (sustenance), desire of search, evolution, welfare and wealth. This is the *chakra* of life-force and takes care of the stomach, intestines, spleen and liver. Its negative aspects are involvement in domestic problems, dominance over spouse, either fasting or excessive interest in food, asceticism, materialism and alcohol. In positive sense, it advocates the ten commandments as the guideline for Self-realisation. *Kundalini* first awakens in *manipur*, piercing it from one extreme to the other. Its presiding deities are Lord Vishnu and Sri Lakshmi, and so, care is taken for physical and material well-being. *Dharma* and stomach seem to be related; whenever one revolts against *dharma*, one's stomach gets upset. *However, after seeing the truth and beauty of the Spirit on awakening, one does not care for worldly things and becomes a witness to the Self. One learns to have faith in Providence, gains strength to take responsibilities and enjoy duties. Interest in alcohol and temptation for special dishes or fasting vanishes, and one's appetite is very easily satisfied. One attains the power to create and destroy worlds through the power of speech. Presence of a saintly person is known to bring a sense of quiet and stillness into a group of tumultuous people. Manipur is at the boundary between physical and spiritual worlds; its awakening normally brings visits to higher realms through astral bodies in dreams, trances or visions.*

The fourth one is the *anahat chakra* (heart centre) located at the spinal centre of the region of heart, with twelve petals and air as its element. *Anahata means unstruck; the awakening of chakra promises the hearing with the inner ear of the Cosmic Sound – Aum or Word, which is created without the striking of two objects; it is heard when all the internal noises of the mind have been stopped through sustained practices. The chakra represents existence, love, truth, and after awakening: truth-attention-joy (Sat-Chit-Ananda).* Its negative aspects are extreme physical and mental activities, bad relations – especially with mother, drugs, no faith in God, anti-God activities. Its presiding deities are Lord Shiva and Sri Parvati, the *Atma* or Spirit. *On awakening, one loses identification with body, mind and feelings, and one really becomes the Spirit or* Atman *because of the open and clean heart. Forgiveness, all-pervading attention and care of Sri Jagadamba – Mother of the Universe – are received. One develops reverence for one's physical mother, who has a place at the left of the heart, and one's father, who has a place at the right of the heart. We realise that we actually choose our parents. Pure love is detached and it gives unconditionally, flowing like a river. Elimination of self-will and removal of self-protective screens enables one to put oneself in another's shoes and understand the person.*

The fifth one is the *vishuddhi chakra* (throat centre) located at the juncture of the spine and medula oblongata, having sixteen petals and ether as its element. It represents collective consciousness, divine attitude, androgynous personality and playful witness. Its presiding deity is Lord Krishna with Sri Radha for the centre of the *chakra*. Lord Krishna is the eternal witness, watching the cosmic drama with complete detachment. The deity of the left side of *chakra* is Lord Krishna's sister Sri Vishnumaya, representing brother-sister relationship on the positive side, and immorality, guilt, sarcastic attitude and foul tongue on the negative side. The deity of the right side of *chakra* is Bala Krishna (Lord Krishna as child), representing witnessing of the Self on the positive side and smoking, problems of cold or bronchial tubes – such as sinus, swearing and chanting on the negative side. Awakening of the *chakra* provides victory over the negative aspects of the left, right and central *chakra* and realisation of all the positive aspects. *Vishuddhi chakra* takes care of the physical parts such as arms, face, throat, mouth and teeth and suggests protection from cold, smoking habits and negligence of dental care. *Awakening promises freedom from "worldly desires", as they have served their purpose by now. The energy hitherto used for achieving worldly goals, is now free and redirected upwards to open the "gateway of liberation". Eternal knowledge from* mooladhara *and wealth of knowledge from* manipur *are combined as the union of subjective and objective at the* vishuddhi *leading to the true meaning of yoga – union. A shift from intellectual to deeper level gives peace of mind and understanding of the past with clarity, seeing the present and anticipating the future. Increased awareness and greater discrimination clearly tell about what should be done and what should be avoided. One becomes merciful to all, knowing that one is a product of one's circumstances and victim of one's own ignorance.*

The sixth one is the *ajna chakra* (eyebrow centre), also known as the "centre of command" or the "third eye". It is located at the centre of the brain, having two petals. The presiding deity of the central *chakra* is Lord Jesus Christ, representing forgiveness and resurrection, that of left chakra is Lord Mahavira representing subconscious (superego) and the deity of right *chakra* is Lord Buddha representing *ahankar* (ego). The positive aspects of the centre are sight, hearing and thought and the negative aspects are bad association and wandering eyes; the positive aspects of the left are memories and conditioning from the past, and the negative aspects are addictions and self-indulgence; the positive aspects of the right are I-ness and the negative aspects are worries, harmful attitude towards others and incorrect notions of God. *Ajna* is supposed to be the most important *chakra* where *ida* and *pinagla* culminate. *With the arrival of* kundalini *on this chakra, thoughtless awareness brings blissful silence which is at the heart of creation; one is in direct communication with the creator and commands are received here. Yogis undergo an experience of death, ego is fragmented into millions of pieces and one enters the state of* shunya *(void) or absolute nothingness. This is one's second birth from mother* Kundalini *with the blessings of Paramashiva. According to the message of Lord Jesus, one is resurrected and born again into a new awareness of the Self.* Karma *is the result of past actions from ego, and oneness with the spirit takes one beyond ego and* karma; *vestiges of imperfection are purified and the* karmas *are burned away. God's compassion is expressed through our forgiveness, and the person forgiven may not be affected but our chains are broken. One is now androgynous,* ardhanareeshwara *– half male, half female, having a perfect balance of intellect and intuition. One knows more than three or four dimensions, which cannot be described, it can only be experienced.*

Compassion, which was expressed earlier only to friends and relatives or dear ones, and later to worthy though unknown people brought to one's attention, is at this stage extended to unsociable, alcoholic, violent and downtrodden, since the compassion has reached the level of Divinity. One begins to feel grateful to even those who have been one's critics and made one's life miserable. However, temptations continue to come even in the life of saints and yogis, but they are more subtle now. The Guru can make a mistake too, but a purpose may not be there. Saints, Gurus or seekers, who are on the wrong path in your opinion, must be put into Light. The *ajna chakra* gives the power of awareness and discrimination, but it should be crowned with compassion.

The three *nadis* – *ida, pingala* and *sushumna* – are represented by three great rivers in mythology: the Ganga, the Jamuna and the Saraswati, respectively. The "*sangam*", that is, the meeting place or the convergence of the three rivers is called "Triveni", near present-day Prayag or Allahabad in India. According to Hindu belief, every twelve years, when the sun is in Aquarius, a dip at the point of confluence purifies the person. The *ajna chakra* is very important and it is symbolically represented by this point of confluence; its awakening signifies expansion of awareness, transcendence of the realm of duality and precipitation of the "stored *karmas*" to the surface, which, when faced and squared with great efforts, transform the person from manhood to Godhood. Women in India apply *sindur* (vermilion) at the exact point of the *ajna chakra,* which was meant to maintain a constant conscious and unconsciousness awareness of the *chakra;* it was not a religious mark or a beauty spot, at it is wrongly understood today. Men in the same way apply *tilak* (paste of sandalwood) at the point of the third eye. The purpose of *sindur* or *tilak* is to exert a constant pressure on the nerve which runs from *bhrumadhyaa* (centre of eyebrows) to the medulla oblongata, which has presently been forgotten. The health of the pineal gland, which is responsible for the development of the *ajna chakra,* can be regenerated and maintained through yogic techniques, such as, *trataka* (concentration in front of the third eye) and *shambhavi mudra.*

A sixth or intuitive sense works through the awakened *ajna chakra,* which also gives rise to the faculty of astral projection and inner visions in the dream state. One is now standing under the *kalpataru* (wish-fulfilment tree) and one's mental resolves in accordance with *dharma* are immediately converted into fruits. One is a detached observer or witness of all events of life and nothing disturbs one. One participates in all affairs of life and lives fully, but as a detached witness. One surrenders and moves freely with the fast moving current of the flowing life. The person has awakened from the dream of life and has already seen one's future in higher realms through dreams and visions.

Regarding two petals of the *chakra,* the left one signifies *ida nadi,* the right one signifies *pingala nadi* and the two of them meet with the central *nadi sushumna;* the merging taking place just below the *ajna chakra.* Letters inscribed on the two petals are *Ham* and *Kshem,* which is the "*bija* (seed) *mantra*" for Shiva and *Shakti.* The importance of *Shivalingam* should now be understood at this point. It is not a phallic symbol but a symbol of one's astral body. *Lingam* in *mooladhara,* called *dhumra lingam*, has a smoky colour, representing the undeveloped state of consciousness with instincts. *Lingam* at the *ajna chakra,* called *Itarakhya lingam,* has a black colour, representing I-awareness and various powers associated with it. *Lingam* in *sahasrara,* called *jyotir lingam,* is luminous, representing illumined state of consciousness. During meditation, consciousness passes from one stage to another: instinctive and restless, calm and quiet, and illumined. The practitioner witnesses the three lingams during the course of his inner journey. Successful arrival at *ajna* is indicated by the realisation of its deity Paramshiva, according to traditional terminology, who shines like a chain of lightning flashes during meditation on *ajna chakra.*

On meditating at the awakened *ajna chakra,* one sees a flaming lamp shining like the morning sun. Results of meditation, on various *chakras,* are collectively realised by meditation on the *ajna chakra* alone. One has realised one's unity with Brahman and certain superpowers (*siddhis*) are acquired by the person according to one's grooming and interest. For example, if a person is a writer, his writings become very effective and powerful through the divine influence. The next and last station is *sahasrara chakra,* which is the culmination of the journey of *kundalini.* However, "it is not important for us to know how to reach *sahasrara* from *ajna chakra,* but it is essential for us to know how to awaken *ajna."* (Saraswati 1984, 142) If *ajna chakra* is awakened before other *chakras,* then none or fewer difficulties are faced by the practitioner. Awakening other *chakras* one by one brings several unprecedented difficulties. Hence, it is highly advisable to concentrate on the *ajna chakra* than on others. Since the *mooladhara chakra* is internally connected to the *ajna chakra,* awakening of *ajna* automatically triggers the awakening of the *mooladhara,* and the opening of other *chakras* also becomes easier.

The seventh one is the *sahasrara chakra* (crown centre) located four fingers-breadth above the crown of the head, having a thousand petals. It represents integration, silence and cosmic consciousness, and is manifested as vibrations and cool breeze. Its positive aspects are going beyond the duality and above the three states of being or *gunas,* called *tamas* (inertia), *rajas* (activity) and *sattva* (purity). Its negative aspect is disbelief in God. Since the location of the *sahasrara* is beyond the physical body, it is not in fact a *chakra.* It is the culmination of the yogic process and crown of expanded awareness signified through the thousand petals. It is Brahman – represented by *shunya* (void) – nothing and everything. Transcending all concepts, it is, nevertheless, source of all concepts. *Arrival of* kundalini *at sahasrara marks the union of Shiva and Shakti and it is the beginning of* samadhi, *that is, Self-realisation. Between* ajna *and* sahasrara *the experience of death, absolute nothingness or* shunyata *(void) and "merging of the seer, seeing and seen" takes place. This is* nirvana, *enlightenment,* nirvikalpa samadhi, *Self-realisation or the Kingdom of God. It is supramental awareness, awareness of one's own Self.*

Awareness is of three kinds: awareness of senses – touch, taste, smell, sound and forms; awareness of mind – time, space and object; supramental awareness, which is a process, a range of experiences – *samadhi. Samadhi* is further classified into three categories by Patanjali: *savikalpa samadhi,* that is *samadhi* with fluctuations; *asampragyata,* that is *samadhi* without awareness; and *nirvikalpa samadhi,* that is *samadhi* without fluctuations. Just as one cannot know when childhood ends and youth begins, and when youth ends and old age begins, even so one cannot know when meditation ends and *samadhi* begins. One cannot pinpoint it, it is an interaction between two states. The whole process occurs in continuity, each state fusing into the next and transforming in a very graduated way. Experiences, when *kundalini* ascends through the various *chakras,* are indicative of the evolving nature of consciousness and they are within the realm of *savikalpa samadhi* – illumination and darkness occurring now and then. At the point of experience of death at the *ajna chakra, savikalpa samadhi* ends and *nirvikalpa samadhi* begins. "From here, energies fuse and flow together to *sahasrara,* where enlightenment unfolds. *Kundalini* awakening and *samadhi* are the same thing. If you understand the teachings of Buddha and other great saints and teachers, you will find that they have all spoken about the same thing but in different languages." (Saraswati 1984, 204-205) Patanjali's *raja yoga* is an intellecutal approach leading to the highest point of *nirvikalpa samadhi,* while *tantra* is an emotional approach leading to the highest point of *sahasrara;* awareness in both cases is the same.

Conclusion and Suggestions

Just as the food in a utensil cannot be cooked over the flame of a candle, even so *kundalini* cannot be awakened through limited amount of prayers or worships. If the utensil is placed over some heating device capable of producing a temperature of 100 degrees, the food will be cooked in a very short time. Even so, if the spiritual pressure of 100 degrees is applied over the *kundalini,* it can be awakened in a single lifetime. Almost all religions of the world have become obsolete since they are not stronger than the flame of a candle. That is why the followers of different religions fight against each other, as the power has not awakened in them and they have not undergone the inner transformation. If Krishna, Buddha, Jesus, Mohammed, Zoroaster, Confucius, Lao Tse, Gurdjief, Mahavira, Nanak and Pythagoras were sitting at a round table, they would have a perfect understanding and love for each other. Each one of them had his "spiritual power" awakened through a device of 100 degrees and they all understood one and the same God. It is a pity that their followers, in general, never know and learn the "method of 100 degrees" and they remain ordinary persons. Of course, there have been and will always be a selected few in each faith who knew the secret and reached the goal.

The secret has been presented in this chapter, which, if followed in the right manner, can awaken the *kundalini* in one lifetime and you can join the band of selected few who know themselves and God. The integral approach covers most of disciplines of development and there is a very little chance, if any, for its failure or for giving rise to abnormalities in a practitioner which are due to one-sided methods. Bronwyn Fox, the Australian researcher and bestselling author of *Panic: Don't Panic,* agreed with me in the 1992 conference in California that the main cause of psychic disorders with which a large number of people in Australia are suffering today, is an uneven way of living and spiritual development. *Kundalini* is an energy of infinite order and it overshoots in the neglected department of development.

In the previous chapter, various possible methods have been discussed. In fact, the methods are not mutually exclusive and perfection of any one path will invariably include elements from many other paths. For example, whatever method one follows, one's stages of development are always seen in dreams. Guides in different faiths have always advised practitioners to pay regular attention to dreams and get advantage from it. Paths of knowledge, devotion and *karma* are usually seen to run parallel in a yogi, some more, some less, and each one is careful about his dreams as well. Most practitioners are married persons and traditional religions tell them to avoid sex which is a sinful act according to them. So the practitioners are in a fix; they want to come out of it but they cannot, so they live with guilt. So whatever path they may be following, they have to know a way to conquer sex. Love, prayer and solitude – each is an independent path in itself. But the fact is, whatever path a practitioner may be following, he has to have intense love since love is God, he has to live in solitude for sufficient periods of time so that the Spirit can interact with the person, and prayer is a part of most disciplines in a natural way. So you see, a large number of disciplines are to be lived simultaneously, and it is for this purpose that *ashrams* were built with the services of an experienced guide. However, if one can have an urge to learn and practise things, one can do without a guide too, although it may take a little longer to get to the goal. And once you reach the goal, it is the same thing for all.

The Point of No Return

God has no life; He is "existence", and it is the experience of this "existence" which is called *samadhi.* Normally, when the "inner atom bomb" blasts, that is, when *kundalini* reaches *sahasrara,* there is a brief experience of "death and resurrection"; one passes through *samadhi* and the experience of Self or God, and then comes back to normal life with a change. The change is that one has a second birth, one is reborn, manhood ends and Godhood begins. But in later encounters, and sometimes even in the first encounter with reality, the person may be absorbed and lost forever; one may not return from the sojourn into normal existence which one had before *samadhi.* One is dead on the physical level, and the translation into higher realm has taken place. This is called "the point of no return". Meher Baba was lost in such a state for four to five days; he did not know what he was wearing or eating or doing. Ramakrishna would go into such a state just by hearing the name of Rama or Krishna, or by seeing a temple or any kind of religious sign.

A great care is needed at such a juncture. Meher Baba was saved because of his disciples ever present there and Ramakrishna was saved primarily because of one of his nephews. Whenever he was going in such a state, his beloved nephew would feed him or give him massage to restore the breathing, according to the situation. The world knows the name of Vivekananda who spread the teachings of Ramakrishna, but nobody knows the name of his nephew who saved his life for the world. Ramakrishna did another thing himself to save himself to carry the message to the world; he maintained a taste for delicious food and new varieties every day. Someone asked him the reason for tasty food and that day his bell was rung. Although he explained that the interest in food was keeping him alive for the world, but then he lost that last interest too on being pointed out about it, and the third or the fourth day he was dead. No one could save him. Unless there is a school, a group or an *ashram* around the practitioner, either one will not be able to go into *samadhi,* or, if once gone into it, one will not be able to get back to normal life. Hence, some kind of organisation is recommended around the person who is likely to go into *samadhi.*

The state of *samadhi* is extremely blissful and it becomes very difficult to cut it short. As I pointed out earlier, one touches this state briefly and comes back. Perhaps this is the design of nature. But on repeated happenings, one fine day, one may be plunged into it not to return again. I can say so with my own experiences, and I am really afraid to go into *samadhi* when I am alone. Of course, one day it will happen, but those who can convey the truth to the world in one way or the other, and those who do not want to leave even this reason behind – because this can be the seed of another incarnation – would like to keep the allotted existence on earth in a natural way. Let me remind here that the rule of "fixed destiny" does not apply on yogis, who are the ones gone beyond the force of gravitation. A yogi makes his own destiny and is free to choose his time of death. There have been innumerable realised souls who are unknown to the world because they had no literary training or could not have an impact with the world, for one reason or the other. And it is the experience of only those who have gone beyond who can tell about what is beyond, to whatever extent it may be possible within the constraints; there is no other source. It is not unusual to find some special interests in the life of saints and prophets or the realised souls, which keeps them alive on earth. Hence, such people should not be criticised on the basis of those special interests and must be preserved as the advocates of truth.

LAST WORDS

I feel, part of the intent and value of this book is in its pointing out the parallel foundations in all orthodox religions. There are always two main paths in a world based on a belief in polarity. These are value judgments such as right and wrong, good and evil and in or out. We can search for mutual peace by exploring all the external dogmatic teachings of the various competing religions and after a comprehensive, explorative comparison of them all, come to the understanding that fundamentally they all demand the same thing. Religion demands adherence. Most of the world's people have been conditioned to believe that chasing after this goal of religious law, outside themselves, will lead to peace, happiness, and ultimately, the experience of a particular definition of Heaven. If only they can convince or coerce every other person on the planet that they are the possessors of the only regulations that are right or that God approves of. There would be peace if only somebody everyone can be taught God's one and only true name, whatever that may be. What religious competitors commonly forget are the two most powerful tenets basic to all scripture, love and compassion, complete spiritual opposites of religious competition and judgment.

There is a reason, despite all the energy expended over thousands of years, that this peace has not yet come about in a lasting way. Peace, happiness, love and Heaven are not found outside of our own hearts. They are in our own being-ness. Love is what we are created of. The people of the world all want the same two things, happiness and an escape from suffering. And as always, there is another method to discover this. The orthodox study and observation of what we *are not* can lead us to what we *are*. This will bring us to the other path.

Cosmic Consciousness is a state already existing and waiting to be uncovered within everyone. Within the state of Cosmic Consciousness, the reality of who we truly are, dawns like the sun dawns each morning. Sunshine comes because it has always been there, only during the night it was hidden in the shadow of the earth's body, just as our fearful beliefs are a dark shadow separating us from our hearts, love and the true nature of all that is. Something similar occurs when we identify ourselves as our bodies and fear their loss will also be the loss of who we feel we are. Our Cosmic Consciousness is overshadowed by our confusion that we are our bodies. Cosmic Consciousness is the direct experience of not only the universe and God's true nature, it is also the experience of our own true beings as well. In that first instant of dawning, the fearful shadow of misunderstanding begins to evaporate before the light of universal love. This is a purely natural phenomenon that cannot be forced or counterfeited and will manifest in all beings at some point in every being's infinite spiritual evolution. Perhaps we can delay its coming by sleepwalking through life, but our ultimate awakening is as inevitable as the birthright of our existence. There is also the strong possibility of encouraging and speeding its coming.

Arousal of Kundalini energy is one way to begin the dawning of Cosmic Consciousness and attain freedom from life after life of experience founded on fear and judgement. This book has the information to assist spiritual aspirants in finding their own path. Cosmic Consciousness lies within us just as the path to realise it also lies within.

Our own life experiences, and those of the people around us, give hints of the Universe's nature, just as dreams and visions show us the possibility of other truths and realities. Near-death experiences, in which the events witnessed are later verified as accurate, and past-life memories that have been verified as true events, are two examples of other realities. The slowing of perceived time during a dangerous crisis can generate an understanding of the illusion of time and the limited truth of the speed of light. Indeed, everything we perceive as reality is fundamentally a quantum event. These types of experiences will lead to a realisation of four basic, unchanging cosmic truths:

1. We exist infinitely with no beginning and no end. We are not born and cannot die.
2. We are part of All that is; and All that is, is within us.
3. The Law of Cause and Effect; what we put out is what we get back, without exception and in the tiniest detail.
4. With the exception of these laws, everything in the Universe is in a constant state of transformation.

A desire for understanding expands awareness, thus creating possibility for expanded experience. Defining and judging contract awareness and deny our natural openness for greater experience. Expansion of awareness can come through an educated desire or with natural spontaneity. A NDE is naturally spontaneous, and a consciously directed out-of-body soul-travel to other places on earth or to the astral realms can be the result of educated desire. The desire for awakening can come as part of the personality drive at birth or evolve slowly over a lifetime of acquiring enough knowledge to discover that awakening exists and is an achievable reality. On the arrival of awakening and Self-Realisation, much of the burden of judgmental, polarised knowledge is released back into the illusion it spawned from. This freedom, so sought after by humankind, is freedom from our own belief in fear and judgment. We are searching for salvation from our own beliefs. God-Realisation is that salvation; and it comes from within. All humankind is ultimately a candidate for Cosmic Consciousness, whether it occurs as a spontaneous event arising out of crisis or is consciously pursued with an open heart. Learning of the commonality in the natural source of the awakening is a conformation for both the spiritually educated, trained student of liberation, and for those in whom the experience is sudden and unexpected.

This book offers a glimpse into the reality of Cosmic Consciousness and a variety of ways to discover that same reality within us. There are also more ways than those detailed here, as always it is up to us to choose our own path. We will always be offered polarity's two pathways, the inner or outer, taking responsibility or giving our responsibility away, going toward what excites us or running from our fears. There need not be confusion over which path is most suitable, as the intention for taking any given path will generate the results.

The mind and body are inter-connected and supportive of one another. Kundalini is a physical energy requiring a physical mind and body to manifest through. A healthy body and clear mind give Kindalini energy a place to work.

One reason we may be embodied in an organic physical form is to have a vehicle to generate the transformation through.

The path to consciousness can be travelled more easily with training, as we are less likely to believe the experiences are hallucinatory or that we are losing our minds. Our own karmic destiny is supplying us with all the tools we need. Each person's life is a constant steam of choice and opportunity. The simple trust that whatever your Soul is providing you with or guiding you toward is the most perfect and most compassionate possible. It is all that your beliefs will allow. This trust in perfection and love will see you through all of life's transformations.

Throughout time, we have had a fascination with "Healing". Usually that idea of healing has been limited to connections with the physical and emotional body, and we have thought of healing as a singular event. We see something as wrong and we want to fix it, to change it from wrong to right. There is another way to view Healing. We live in a time-stream of existence. In the same way that we view a river as a whole entity composed of several elements, the stream of existence is composed of elements such as love, compassion, peace and Healing, and is eternally flowing. Every moment we are in a constant state of Healing. Perhaps what we are in physical bodies to heal may not actually be our bodies at all. Maybe we arc experiencing ourselves as physical to give a reference point for our consciousness to realise the only thing we can truly heal is our fearful beliefs. The rising of Kundalini and subsequent expansion of awareness are powerful tools in our ability to heal and spiritually evolve. The healing of fear and separation, and spiritual evolution are mutually dependent. Kundalini is an energy of clarity. There may be much opportunity for confusion as it rises in partial stages, but when fully risen, the ability to clearly focus and to understand the underlying and unified compassionate nature of reality dawns with the clear light of the Soul.

Jonathan Barber

BIBLIOGRAPHY

Agarwal, Rahul, 1997. "Martial Arts is a way of Life". *The Hindustan Times*, New Delhi, October 22, 1997.

Asaramji, Saint, 1994. *Sachcha Sukh*. Saint Asaramji Ashram, Sabarmati, Ahmedabad, India.

Atwater, P. M. H., 1988. *Coming Back to Life*. New York: Dodd, Mead.

Aurobindo, Sri, 1970. *The Life Divine*. Sabda, Sri Aurobindo Ashram, Pondicherry, India.

_______, n.d. 2, *The Synthesis of Yoga*. Sabda, Sri Aurobindo Ashram, Pondicherry, India.

_______, n.d. 3, *Savitri*. Sabda, Sri Aurobindo Ashram, Pondicherry, India.

_______, 1958. *Letters on Yoga*. Sabda, Sri Aurobindo Ashram, Pondicherry, India.

_______, 1982. *Thoughts and Aphorisms*. Sri Aurobindo Ashram, Pondicherry, India.

_______, 1986. *The Yoga of Divine Works – Karmayoga*. Sri Aurobindo Ashram, Pondicherry, India.

_______, and The Mother, 1989. *The Psychic Being*. Sri Aurobindo Ashram, Pondicherry, India.

Baba, Meher, 1967. *Discourses by Meher Baba Vol. I, II, III*. Sufism Reoriented Inc., San Francisco.

Bancroft, Anne, 1976. *Twentieth-Century Mystics and Sages.* Penguin Group, London.

Besant, Annie, 1923. *Initiation: The Perfecting of Man.* Chicago, IL: Theosophical Press.

________, 1966. *Death – And After.* The Theosophical Publishing House, Madras, India.

Beversluis, Joel, 1995. *A Source Book for Earth's Community of Religions.* Grand Rapids, MI: CoNexus Press & NY: Global Ed. Associates.

Blavatsky, Helena P., 1980-1988. *Collected Writings.* Vol. 1-16, Wheaton, IL: Theosophical Publishing House.

Borgia, Anthony, n.d. *More About Life in the World Unseen.* Uddam Press Ltd., London, UK.

Bucke, R. M., 1961. *Cosmic Consciousness.* The Citadel Press, Secaucus, New Jersey.

Chakrapani, 1997. "Chamatkar Hi Tha Vah". *Manohar Kahanian,* 281 Mutthiganj, Allahabad, India, March 1997.

________, 1997. "Trikal Siddhi". *Manohar Kahanian* 281, Mutthiganj, Allahabad, India, May 1997.

Chatterji, Mohini M., 1932. *Vivek-Chudamani* or *The Crest – Jewel of Wisdom of Sri Sankaracharya.* TPS, Adyar, Madras, India.

Dalal, Nergis, 1998. "Towards a Higher Awareness". *The Hindustan Times,* New Delhi, March 23, 1998.

David-Neel, Alaxandra, 1931. *Mystere et Magique en Tibet.* France.

Dey, A. K., n.d. *Khajuraho – The Immortal Ancient Sculpture.* Jayna Publishing Co., Delhi.

Field, Rashid, 1976. *The Last Barrier.* Harper & Row Publishers, NY.

Globe, Diane, 1993. *Through the Tunnel.* S.O.U.L. Foundation, Palm Harbor, Florida.

Goswami, Amit with Richard E. Reed and Maggie Goswami, 1993. *The Self-Aware Universe.* NY: Jeremy P. Tarcher / Putnam Book, G. P. Putnam's Sons.

Goyal, J. D., 1996. *Mrityu Ke Bad (Occult Science).* Hind Pocket Books, New Delhi.

Guiley, Rosemary Ellen, 1991. *Harper's Encylopedia of Mystical and Paranormal Experiences.* Harper, San Francisco.

Haich, Elisabeth, 1982. *Sexual Energy and Yoga.* Arora Press, New York, NY 10003.

Hall, Manly P., 1928. *An Encyclopaedic Outline of Masonic, Hermetic, Qabbalistic and Rosicrucian Symbolican Philosophy.* H. S. Crocker Co., San Francisco.

Hamid, A., 1997. "Ma Ka Dil". *Manohar Kahanian,* 281 Mutthiganj, Allahabad, India, March 1997.

Haridass, Baba, 1980. *From Sweeper to Saint.* Sri Ram Publishing, Santa Cruz, California.

Haslop, F., n.d. *Life Worth Living.* Brook House, 23 Warwick Lane, London, UK.

Herbert, Nick, 1987. *Quantum Reality.* Anchor Books, NY: Double Day.

Huxley, Aldous, 1944. *The Perennial Philosophy.* Harper & Row Publishers, NY.

Jain, P. K., 1997. "God-less Karma for Salvation". *The Hindustan Times,* New Delhi, September 15, 1997.

James, Ivor, 1996. *The Astral World.* Audio Tape, London, UK.

Jayaram, Amit, 1997. "Meditations: Freedom From Choice". *The Hindustan Times,* New Delhi, September 22, 1997.

Jung, C. G., n.d. 1. *The Collected Works.*

________, n.d. 2 *The Psychological Types.*

________, 1961. *Memories, Dreams, Reflections;* recorded and edited by Aniela Jaffe NY: Random House.

_______, 1964. *Man and His Symbols*. Double Day & Co., New York.

Khan, Maulana Wahiduddin, 1998 "Pilgrimage – Highest Form of Worship". *The Hindustan Times*, New Delhi, March 30, 1998.

Klemp, Herald, 1987. *Soul Travellers of the Far Country*. Eckankar, Minneapolis, MN.

Krishna, Gopi, 1975. *The Awakening of Kundalini*. Kundalini Research Foundation, New York.

Kumar, Ravindra, 1992. *Secrets of Numerology*. Sterling Publishers Pvt. Ltd., New Delhi.

_______, 1994. *Journey Back Home, Part IV, Personality Transformation with Chakras*. JRPR, Oct. 1994.

_______, 1997. *Destiny, Science and Spiritual Awakening*. Sterling Publishers Pvt. Ltd., New Delhi.

_______, 1997. *Psychic Individuation and Self-Realization – I*. JRPR, July 1997.

_______, 1998. *Journey Back To Our True Home – Through Spiritual Energy Kundalini*. Emberlight Publishers, Florida.

Kvastad, Nils Bjorn, 1980. *Problems of Mysticism*. Scintilla Press, Oslo.

Larsson, Erik Gerner, 1963. *Martinus*. Martinus Institute, Copenhagen.

Leadbeater, C. W., 1933. *The Astral Plane*. The Theosophical Publishing House, Madras, India.

Lello, Ronald, S., 1985. *Revelations – Glimpses of Reality*. Shephard-Walwyn Ltd., London.

Long, Max Freedom, 1965. *The Huna Code in Religions*. Huna Research Publications, California.

Martin, Joel and Romanowski, Patricia, 1991. *We Are Not Forgotten*. New York: Berely Books.

Martinus, 1933. *The Fate of Mankind*. Martinus Institute, Copenhagen. (Translated in English in 1986.)

Mehta, Pundrik C., 1994. *The Fundamentals of Indian Philosophy.* A correspondence course, Hindu University, Florida.

Moody, Raymond A. Jr., 1975. *Life After Life.* Bantam Books, New York.

Morris, R. L. & Edge, M. L., 1986. *Foundations of Parapsychology.* Routledge and Kegan Paul, p.l.c., Boston.

Muktananda, Swami, 1972. *Chitshakti Vilas (The Play of Consciousness).* Gurudev Siddhapeeth, Maharashtra, India.

_______, 1979. *Kundalini – The Secret of Life.* Gurudev Siddha Peeth, Ganeshpuri, India.

Myers, W. W. Frederic, 1954. *Human Personality and Its Survival After Death.* Vol. 1 & 2, Longmans, Green & Co., New York.

O'Brien, Stephen, 1989. *Visions of Another World.* The Acquarian Press, London, UK.

O'Brien, Stephan, 1991. *Voices From Heaven.* The Acquarian Press, London, UK.

Pike, James, n.d. *The Other Side.* W. H. Alan, London, UK.

Poddar, Hanumanprasad, n.d. *The Philosophy of Love.*

Radha, Swami Sivananda, 1992. *Kundalini Yoga.* Motilal Banarsidass Publishers, Delhi.

Rajneesh, Osho, 1997. *Kundalini: In Search of the Miraculous.* Sterling Publishers Pvt. Ltd., New Delhi.

Rajneesh, Osho, n.d. *From Sex to Superconsciousness.* The Rebel Publishing House GmbH, Cologne, Germany.

Rao, M. Rajeshwar, n.d. *The Legend of Shri Shirdi Sai Baba and His Teachings.* Sri Sai Baba Mandir, Secunderabad, India.

Reed, Henry, 1995. *Recovering Spirituality from Dreaming – Venture Inward.* A.R.E. Edgar Cayce Foundation, Atlantic University. Sept./Oct. 1995.

Riffel, Herman, 1981. *Your Dreams: God's Neglected Gift.* Ballantine Books, New York.

Rocher, Grace, n.d. *Beyond the Horizon.* Messrs James Clark & Co., 33 Store St., London, UK.

Sahai, Chaturbhuj, 1987. *Sadhana Ke Anubhava.* Ramashraya Satsang, Mathura, India.

________, 1990. *Saint Sri Mira Bai.* Ramashraya Satsanga, Mathura, India.

Satprem, 1985. *On the Way to Supermanhood.* USA: Institute For Evolutionary Research, 200 Park Av. # 303 E, NY 10166.

______, n.d. *Sri Aurobindo on The Adventures of Consciousness.*

Sherwood, Jane, n.d. *Post Mortem Journal.* Messrs Naville Spairman Ltd., 112, Whitefield St., London, UK.

Singh, Satya Prakash, 1986. *Sri Aurobindo and Jung.* Madhucchandas, Aligarh, India.

Sted, W. T., 1897. *After Death.* Tenth ed. 1921. London, UK.

Steiger, Brad, n.d. *In My Soul I am Free.*

Storr, Anthony, 1988. *Solitude – A Return to the Self.* Ballantine Books, New York.

Svoboda, Robert E., 1994. *Kundalini.* Rupa & Co., New Delhi.

Swain, Jasper, 1974. *On the Death of My Son.* Turnstone Books, London, UK.

Tirtha, Vishnu, 1993. *Devatma Shakti (Kundalini) – Divine Power.* Yogashree Peeth Trust, Muni-Ki-Reti (Rishikesh), India.

Twitchell, Paul, 1969. *Eckankar: The Key to Secret Worlds.* San Diego: Illumined Way Press, USA.

Walker, Claire G., 1997. *The Psychic Revolution of the 20th Century and Our Psychic Sense.* Psychic Sense Publishers, 14001 Thunderbird Drive 4K, Seal Beach, CA.

Wangchuk, Sonam, 1998. "The Beauty of Bhavana". *The Hindustan Times,* New Delhi, May 11, 1998.

Woodroffe, Sir John, 1981. *The Serpent Power.* Ganesh & Co., Madras, India.

Yogananda, Paramahansa, 1986. *Autobiography of a Yogi.* Jaico Publishing House, New Delhi.

Zaleski, Carol, 1987. *Other World Journeys: Accounts of Near-Death Experience in Medieval and Modern Times.* New York: Oxford University Press.

Zemke, Leroy E., 1996. *Thoughts For Transformation.* Emberlight Publishers, Florida.

Zukav, Gary, 1989. *The Seat of the Soul.* NY: Fireside Book, Simon & Schuster.

GLOSSARY

Achara dharma	:	Ethical discipline
Adattadana Viramana	:	To accept not when not rightly bestowed
Adi	:	The beginning
Adi lok	:	Plane in the beginning
Agun	:	Absolute, without attributes
Ahankar	:	Ego
Ahimsa	:	Non-injury to others
Ajna chakra	:	Eyebrow centre
Akashik elements	:	Etheric substance
Anahata chakra	:	Heart centre
Ananda	:	Bliss
Anandamaya kosh	:	Unconscious/transcendental dimension
Annamaya kosh	:	Physical body
Anupama	:	Having no parallel
Ardhanareeshwara	:	Half male – half female, Shiva and *Shakti* in one, representing balance of masculinity and feminity
Asampragyata	:	*Samadhi* without awareness
Asanas	:	Yogic postures
Ashram	:	Place of yogic practices
Atman	:	Soul or Spirit, the pure Self, beyond body and mind
Atmic	:	Pertaining to *Atman* or Soul or Spirit
Bal Krishna	:	Lord Krishna as a child

Bhairavi	:	A female tantric deity
Bhakti	:	Devotion
Bhakti sutras	:	Elements of bhakti
Bhakti Yoga	:	The path of devotion
Bhajan	:	Religious song
Bhoga	:	Worldly pleasures
Bhulok	:	Physical plane
Bhrumadhya	:	Eyebrow centre
Bhuvarlok	:	Astral plane, next to the physical plane
Brahmachari	:	Celibate
Buddhic	:	Intellectual
Chakras	:	Seven centres or vortices of energy on the spine
Chaitya purusa	:	Psychic being
Chhaya sharira	:	Etheric double
Comatose torpor	:	A dull trance, defined by Sri Aurobindo
Darshan	:	Seeing in person
Devachan	:	Heaven
Devarsi	:	Superior amongst all *devas* (gods)
Dharma	:	Social or religious discipline
Dharmshala	:	A resting place, hotel or motel
Dristi	:	Direct sight
Dukha	:	Misery, pain or suffering
Durga	:	The benevolent female deity, sitting on a tiger, representing wisdom and power; symbol of the awakened and controlled *Kundalini*
Eckankar	:	The religion of Light and Sound, Minneapolis, MN
Girdharilalji	:	A name of Lord Krishna
Golok	:	Plane of God
Grahastha	:	Householder
Gunas	:	Virtues
Hatha Yoga	:	The path of physical yogic practices, which includes *asanas* (postures), *pranayama* (breath control), *kriyas* (cleansing practices), *bandhas* (locks) and *mudras* (seals)

Hiranyalok	:	A particular division of the astral plane representing the womb of consciousness
Ida	:	Moon channel running to the left of *sushumna*
Jalandhar bandh	:	Throat lock
Japa	:	Chanting of names
Jivatma	:	*Atman*, Soul
Jnana lok	:	Plane of wisdom
Jnana Yoga	:	The path of knowledge
Kali	:	Ferocious goddess, killer of demons, representing freshly awakened and untamed *Kundalini*
Kalpataru	:	Wish-fulfilment tree
Kamalok	:	Plane of desires
Kamakhya Devi	:	Goddess of sexual power/energy
Kanhaiya	:	Another name for Lord Krishna
Karana sharira	:	Causal body
Karma Yoga	:	The path of selfless action; acting without attachment to the fruits or results of one's actions
Khechri mudra	:	Reverting back of the tongue and its rising towards the palate
Kirtan	:	Singing the glories of God
Krodha	:	Anger
Kshem	:	Safety of one's possessions
Kundalini	:	Also known as the Serpent Power or *Shakti*; it is the Creative Cosmic Energy, the female counterpart of God Unmanifested. It belongs to the causal plane, hence it is invisible on the physical plane. It lies dormant at the base of the spine. In human beings only 15 to 20 % of the brain is at work, the rest is asleep; consequently, people live only mediocre life. When *Kundalini* awakens, the brain begins to work more than 20 % and paranormal powers/experiences begin to show up. Finally, it leads to

		evolution and Self/God-realisation
Kundalini Yoga	:	The yoga system specially designed for the awakening of *Kundalini*
Lakshmi	:	Consort of Lord Vishnu, and goddess of wealth
Lobha	:	Greed
Maan	:	Pride
Mahapurusha	:	Great Soul, who has realised God
Maharlok	:	Upper division of mental plane
Maharsi	:	Greatest amongst the rishis
Maithuna viramana	:	To desist from sex
Manasik lok	:	Mental plane
Mandala	:	Psychic pictures
Manipura chakra	:	Naval centre
Maya	:	Illusion, deceit
Mirsavada viramana	:	To desist from telling a lie
Moksha	:	Liberation, nirvana
Monad	:	Spark of God
Monadic	:	Pertaining to monad, the first manifestation of Unmanifest
Muladhara chakra	:	Root centre
Mul-bandh	:	Root lock
Mudras	:	Yogic postures
Naad	:	Internal cosmic sound
Nadis	:	Channels of energy running throughout the body for its nourishment and maintainance
Namaz	:	Prayers prescribed by the Islamic law, to be performed five times daily
Narad Muni	:	A devotee saint of Lord Narayana, who used to travel to different planes by appearing and disappearing at will
Narayana	:	God, Lord Krishna
Nirguna Brahman	:	Brahman without attributes
Nirodha	:	Renunciation
Nirvana	:	Liberation from the cycle of death and rebirth
Nirvichar samadhi	:	Thoughtless awareness
Nirvikalpa samadhi	:	*Samadhi* without fluctuations
Padmasana	:	Lotus posture

Paramatma	:	Supersoul; God
Paramashiva	:	Lord Shiva
Parigraha parimana	:	To fix the size of acquisition
Parvati	:	Consort of Lord Shiva
Pingla	:	Sun channel running to the right of *sushumna*
Prana	:	Cosmic life energy
Pranamaya kosh	:	Etheric double; conscious dimension
Pranayama	:	Deep breathing and breath control
Pranatipata viramana	:	To desist from killing
Pretlok	:	The plane of ghosts and spirits
Purusa	:	Psychic being
Radha	:	Consort of Lord Krishna
Raja	:	King
Raja Yoga	:	Kingly path, superior to all other kinds of yoga, postulated by Patanjali. Beginning with the stability of mind, it takes the practitioner to the highest state of *samadhi*
Rajayogi	:	One devoted to the path of *Raja Yoga*
Rajasic	:	Belonging to activity
Rajogun	:	Properties of action/activities
Ras lila	:	A group dance
Rig Veda	:	Of the four Vedas, Rig Veda is devoted to the path of *jnana yoga*
Rishis	:	Yogic masters of ancient times
Rooh-vatavajjah	:	The Ray of God; Creative energy *Kundalini*
Ruha	:	Soul, Spirit, *Atman*
Satchidananda	:	*Sat-chit-ananda*, Existence knowledge-bliss
Sadachara	:	Right conduct
Sadhana	:	Yogic practice
Sadhu	:	Monk
Sadhvi	:	Nun
Saguna	:	Divine manifestation of God with attributes
Sahasrara	:	Crown centre
Salokya	:	Residence in the abode of God
Samadhi	:	Deep absorption

Sama Veda	:	Of the four Vedas, Sama Veda is devoted to the path of *bhakti yoga*
Samipya	:	Living in close proximity to the Lord
Samyaka-charitra	:	Right conduct
Samyaka-darshan	:	Right belief
Samyaka-jnana	:	Right knowledge
Sangam	:	Meeting point of three rivers – Ganga, Yamuna and Saraswati
Sankalpa	:	Will
Sankatamochan Mahavirji	:	Monkey-God Hanuman
Sankhya	:	Classification of all that is known, without reference to God. The ancient scientific philosophy of India
Sanyasa	:	Renunciation
Saripya	:	Having form similar to Lord
Saraswati	:	Goddess of wisdom
Sarsti	:	Enjoying the same powers as the Lord
Satguru	:	The inner guru, spiritual teacher or guru
Satoguna	:	Properties of purity
Satsanga	:	Company of religious or God-intoxicated people
Sattvic	:	Belonging to purity
Satya lok	:	Plane of Truth
Savikalpa samadhi	:	Samadhi with fluctuations
Sayujjya	:	Absolute identity with Lord
Shabda	:	Internal cosmic sound
Shakti	:	Female counterpart of God, the Creative Energy
Shaktipat	:	Direct transmission of spiritual power by a guru
Shambhavi mudra	:	Gazing at the eyebrow centre
Shunyata	:	Void
Siddha	:	Adept
Siddhi	:	Paranormal or superpowers
Sindur	:	Vermilion
Smriti	:	Inspired memory of Truth
Sravaka	:	Layman
Sravika	:	Laywoman
Sruti	:	Direct hearing

Sthool lok	Physical plane
Sthool sharira	Physical body
Sukha	Comfort, happiness
Sukshma sharira	Astral body
Surati	Creative energy *Kundalini*
Sushumna	The central channel, pathway of the awakened *Kundalini*
Swadhishthan chakra	Pelvic centre
Swargalok	Heaven, lower division of mental plane
Swayambhu linga	The pillar (*linga*) around which *Kundalini* remains coiled in three-and-a-half rounds, closing the opening of the *linga* with its mouth
Tamasic	Belonging to inertia
Tamoguna	Properties of inertia
Tantra Yoga	The path leading to the union of Shiva and *Shakti*, or the masculine and feminine forces, resulting in liberation; using different kinds of yoga, rituals, worship, discipline, meditation and attainment of powers
Tap lok	Plane of austerities
Tapas	Will of the transcendent spirit, defined by Sri Aurobindo
Tat-tvam-asi	That-thou-art
Tilak	Sandalwood paste applied at eyebrow centre by men
Trataka	Concentration in front of third eye
Trikal siddhi	Power to control the past, present and future
Triveni	Place of convergence of three rivers – Ganga, Yamuna and Saraswati, situated in Allahabad, India
Tulpa	Monkey, created through the power of mind, by Alexandra David-Neel
Twice-born	One who is spiritually awakened and liberated
Uddiyan bandh	Navel lock

Upasana	:	Absorption of practitioner in one's own consciousness
Vaikunth lok	:	Plane of God
Vanaprasthi	:	Belonging to the part of life, after married life is completed
Varna	:	Caste or division of society one belongs to
Vasana sharira	:	Astral body
Vasudeva	:	Lord Krishna
Vigyanmaya kosh	:	Subconscious or unconscious dimension; intuitive aspects
Vipassana	:	A particular kind of meditation
Vishnumaya	:	Sister of Lord Krishna
Vishuddhi chakra	:	Throat centre
Yajna	:	Sacrifice on the sacred fire
Yajur Veda	:	Of the four Vedas, Yajur Veda is devoted to the path of *karma yoga*
Yog	:	Providing the needs
Yoga	:	Divine unity of Soul and Supersoul
Yogi	:	One who takes to the discipline of yoga

INDEX

B

C

F

G

H

Q

X

W